NATURAL RELIEF FROM HEADACHES, INSOMNIA & STRESS

Natural Relief from Headaches, Insomnia & Stress

Safe, Effective Herbal Remedies

David Hoffmann

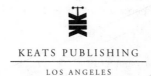

KEATS PUBLISHING

LOS ANGELES

NTC/Contemporary Publishing Group

Library of Congress Cataloging-in-Publication Data

Hoffmann, David, 1951-
    Natural relief from headaches, insomnia, and stress: safe, effective
herbal remedies / by David Hoffmann.
        p. cm.
    Includes bibliographical references and index.
    ISBN 0-87983-982-1
    1. Headache—Alternative treatment. Insomnia—Alternative treatment.
Stress management. 4. Herbs—Therapeutic use.
I. Title.
RC392.H64 1999   99-25559
616. 8'49106—dc21   CIP

Design by Barbara Briggs Garibay

Published by Keats Publishing
A division of NTC/Contemporary Publishing Group, Inc.
4255 West Touhy Avenue
Lincolnwood (Chicago), Illinois 60646-1975 U.S.A.

Printed in the United States of America

International Standard Book Number: 0-87983-982-1

99 00 01 02 03 04 RRD 18 17 16 15 14 13 12 11 10 9 8 7 6 5 4 3 2 1

CONTENTS

A profoundly stressful transformation is affecting all aspects of our culture, often manifesting as trauma, sleep disorders, pain, disruption—the whole panoply of crises we are all too familiar with.

How does one cope with the ever-mounting pressures on our lives in these crazy times? Much has been written about how to manage stress, and much of it contains valuable insights. However, it can be said that at the core of our personal and planetary challenges in the human experience of alienation is a profound spiritual "homesickness." Is there a way in which stress management programs can help us experience the elusive but nurturing sense of belonging?

Herbalism is the medicine of belonging, the direct experience of the whole healing the part. Our world blesses us with herbs, with leaves of life. In the face of humanity's blind abuse and rape of nature, we discover remedies that can help us survive the impact of our mistakes.

Herbalism abounds with opportunities to experience the reality of the healing presence of nature, whether in treating disease or in hugging a tree. Approaching herbalism from its array of diverse and divergent components illuminates a field of human endeavor that is a wonderful weaving of the miraculous and the mundane. It is a therapy that encompasses depression-lifting herbs such as St. John's wort, the spiritual ecstasy of the Amazonian shaman, and the beauty of the flower. The limits to what might be called the path of the herbalist are only those imposed by a parochial vision or imagination!

Herbalism offers the unique possibility of being introduced to our medicine. A bridge can be built between person and herb, empowering the individual to be present and responsible in the healing process. A person can be given a packet of herb seeds, encouraging a direct experience of the life of the plant. This experience of herbal vitality will be translated into a deeper rapport with the impersonal medicine ingested. The patient will not only get the medical benefit from the herb but also the enlivening experience of growing and preparing his or her own healing. If there is no garden, part of the treatment might involve a window box.

Healing with herbal medicines is a unique and wonderful cooperation between humanity and the plants. This experience of wholeness is spirit in action, creating an opportunity for change and transformation. The plant world provides us with herbs that transform and enlighten, and also with plants that heal and nurture nerve tissue itself.

Orthodox medicine tends to reduce psychological problems to a biochemical level and assumes that "appropriate" drugs will sort out or at least hide the problem sufficiently to allow "normal" life to continue. Interestingly enough, some techniques in the field of complementary medicine assume or imply the other extreme: namely, that psychological factors are the cause of all disease. Treatment of the psyche is, therefore, the only appropriate way of healing and will take care of any physical problem. By bringing these two reductionist views together, we come closer to a holistic approach.

A holistic approach to healing acknowledges the interconnectedness of physiological and psychological factors, and regards the nervous system and its functions as a vital element in the treatment of the whole being. To be truly healthy, we have to take care of our physical health through the right diet and lifestyle, but we are also responsible for taking care of our emotional, mental, and spiritual life. We should endeavor to live in a fulfilling, nurturing environment that supports emotional stability. Our thoughts should be creative and life-enhancing, open to the free flow of intuition and imagination, rather than conceptually rigid. And we should stay open to the free flow of the higher energies of our souls, without which health is impossible.

The whole therapy of herbalism is uniquely suited to treating stress, headaches, and sleep disorders. From one perspective, herbs are embodiments of energy and spirit, while from another, they are packets of biochemicals. In fact, they can be viewed as a reflection of the human mind/brain itself! If used with awareness, it is possible to address the needs of the human energy body as well as the tissue involved. In fact, the complexities of the mind/body actually can help the herbalist select the correct remedy. Herbal medicine can be an ecologically and spiritually integrative tool—an ideal counterpart on the physical level for therapeutic techniques on the psychological level.

PART I

Headaches

1

What Are Headaches and What Causes Them?

Headaches, one of the most common health problems affecting humanity, are among the ten most common symptoms for which medical advice is sought, accounting for 18 million outpatient visits a year in the United States. More than 40 million Americans suffer from chronic headaches without regard to race, culture, lifestyle, occupation, or geography. For at least half of these people, the problem is severe and sometimes disabling. In addition to loss of productivity, billions of dollars are spent on various forms of treatment and habituation to medications, plus the significant resulting family and work problems. Despite their prevalence, headaches aren't simply the by-product of a modern, fast-paced society. Medical records left by ancient cultures from the Orient to the New World describe headaches.

Why Does It Hurt?

What hurts in a headache? Several areas of the head can hurt, including those affected by a network of nerves extending over the scalp and by certain nerves in the face, mouth, and throat. Also sensitive to pain, because they contain delicate nerve fibers, are the muscles of the head and blood vessels found along the surface and at the base of the brain. The bones of the skull and tissues of the brain itself, however, never hurt because they lack pain-sensitive nerve fibers.

Pain is a complex experience consisting of a physiological response to a "painful" stimulus followed by an emotional response. It is a warning mechanism that helps to protect us and is primarily associated with injury, or the threat of injury, to bodily tissues. But headache pain is different. For most headaches, even when the pain is severe, there is no underlying disease—not even a brain tumor.

The point at which a stimulus begins to become painful is the pain perception threshold; most studies have found this point to be relatively similar among disparate groups. However, the pain tolerance threshold, the point at which pain becomes unbearable, varies significantly. Childhood experiences, cultural attitudes, genetic makeup, and gender are factors that contribute to the development of each individual's perception of and response to different types of pain. Although some people may be able to physiologically withstand pain better than others, cultural factors rather than heredity usually account for this ability.

Your head can ache in a variety of ways:

- **Severity.** The pain can range from mild to excruciating, annoying to incapacitating.
- **Frequency and duration.** It can strike occasionally or daily, lasting a few minutes to hours or days.
- **Related symptoms.** It can be accompanied by other problems, such as nausea or vomiting.
- **Location.** The pain can be localized in one spot or it can affect the entire head.

When to Have Your Headaches Evaluated

About 90 percent of all headaches are *not* caused by a serious disorder and can be treated effectively with herbal pain relievers alone or in combination with rest, ice packs, or a variety of relaxation techniques. However, there are certain symptoms that should be regarded as indicators that a competent medical diagnosis is called for. These include:

- Sudden, severe headache.
- Headache associated with convulsions.
- Headache accompanied by confusion or loss of consciousness.
- Headache following a blow to the head.
- Headache associated with pain in the eye or ear.
- Persistent headache in a person who was previously headache-free.
- Recurring headache in children.
- Headache that interferes with normal life.
- Headache that occurs three or more times per week.
- Headache that worsens over a period of weeks or months.
- Headache following a head or neck injury.
- Headache that begins after age fifty.
- Headache accompanied by blurred vision or slurred speech, numbness, weakness, or loss of feeling in a limb.
- Headache accompanied by confusion or drowsiness.
- Headache accompanied by fever, nausea, shortness of breath or vomiting, and/or unexpected symptoms that affect the eyes, ears, nose, or throat.

- Headache precipitated by exertion such as exercise, coughing, sneezing, or bending over.

Kinds of Headaches

Headaches brought on by muscle spasms are classified as tension headaches; those caused by the dilation of blood vessels are called vascular headaches. A more specialized classification by the International Headache Society further divides headaches into fourteen categories. A system that helps the herbalist select the appropriate remedy divides headaches into these groupings:

- **Environmental.** Caused by pollutants, body posture, lighting, sound, etc.
- **Stress.** Physical, emotional, or mental upset.
- **Dietary.** Possible allergy to certain foods, medications, or additives, e.g., xanthine-containing foods.
- **Organic.** Caused by a disease such as hypertension.

Pain may also be referred to the head (i.e., felt in the head even though the site of the disease is elsewhere) by eye disorders such as glaucoma and refractive errors, infections or tumors of the nasal sinuses, dental infections, and arthritis of the neck.

Muscle Contraction and Tension Headaches

These are continuous and generalized pains felt from front to back or all around the head and are generally less severe than migraines. The pain is usually a dull ache that has been described as feeling like a tight band around the head. A tension headache can be simply a feeling of pressure or severe enough to cause painful knots in the neck and scalp muscles.

While emotional stress and letdown after such stress are the most common causes, arthritis of the joints of the neck may also contribute. Tension headaches alone are also often experienced by migraine sufferers, and a combined form of headache can also occur.

Tension headache is named not only for the role of stress in triggering the pain but also for the contraction of neck, face, and scalp muscles brought on by stressful events. Tension headache is a severe but temporary form of muscle contraction headache. The headache usually disappears after the period of stress is over.

By contrast, chronic muscle contraction headaches can last for weeks, months, and sometimes years. The pain of these headaches is often described as a tight band around the head or a feeling that the head and neck are in a cast. The pain is steady and is usually felt on both sides of the head. Chronic muscle contraction headaches can cause sore scalps; even combing one's hair can be painful.

Occasionally, muscle contraction headaches are accompanied by nausea, vomiting, and blurred vision, but there is no preheadache syndrome as with migraine. Muscle contraction headaches have not been linked to hormones or foods, as has migraine, nor is there a strong hereditary connection.

For many people, chronic muscle contraction headaches are caused by depression and anxiety. These people tend to get their headaches in the early morning or evening when conflicts in the office or home are anticipated. Depression and anxiety have also been noted to lower both the pain perception and pain tolerance thresholds; anger or excitement, however, can obscure or lessen pain temporarily.

Emotional factors are not the only triggers of muscle-contracting headaches. Certain physical postures—such as holding one's chin down while reading—can lead to head and neck pain. Tensing head and neck muscles during sexual excitement can also cause headache. So can prolonged writing under poor light, holding a phone between the shoulder and ear, or even gum chewing.

More serious problems that can cause muscle contraction headaches include degenerative arthritis of the neck and temporomandibular joint dysfunction or TMJ. TMJ is a disorder of the joint between the temporal bone (above the ear) and the mandible or lower jawbone. The disorder results from poor bite and jaw clenching.

Treatment of muscle contraction headaches varies. The first consideration is to treat any specific disorder or disease that may be causing the headache. For example, arthritis of the neck is treated with anti-inflammatory herbs, and TMJ may be helped by corrective devices for the mouth and jaw. People who suffer infrequent muscle contraction headaches may benefit from a hot shower or moist heat applied to the back of the neck. Cervical collars are sometimes recommended as an aid to good posture. Physical therapy, massage, and gentle exercise of the neck may also be helpful.

Vascular Headaches

Vascular headaches are so named because they are thought to involve abnormal function of the brain's blood vessels or vascular system. These include migraine and its variants as well as headaches due to abnormal stretching of the arterial walls in the cranium as a result of vessel-wall disease.

MIGRAINE

Migraine is an all-too-common problem today. A recent study suggests that 8.7 million women and 2.6 million men suffer from migraine with moderate to severe disability. Of these, 3.4 million women and 1.1 million men experience one or more attacks a month.

Orthodox medicine holds that the fundamental cause of migraine is unknown. The herbalist, as with most holistically orientated practitioners, can achieve excellent results with migraine by focusing on a number of factors that suggest causal links. Specific herbal remedies can prove exceptionally successful if used in the context of addressing the whole body and environment of the patient.

Although the precise cause of migraine headaches is unknown, a key element is flood flow changes in the brain. People who get migraine headaches appear to have blood vessels that overreact to various triggers. One theory that might explain these changes suggests that the nervous system responds to a trigger by creating a spasm in the nerve-rich arteries at the base of the brain. The spasm closes down or constricts several arteries supplying blood to the brain, including the scalp artery and the carotid or neck arteries. As these arteries constrict, the flow of blood to the brain is reduced. At the same time, blood-clotting particles called platelets clump together, a process that is believed to release a chemical called serotonin. Serotonin acts as a powerful constrictor of arteries, further reducing the blood supply to the brain. Reduced blood flow decreases the brain's supply of oxygen. Symptoms signaling a headache, such as distorted vision or speech, may then result.

Reacting to the reduced oxygen supply, certain arteries within the brain open wider to meet the brain's energy needs. This widening or dilation spreads, finally affecting the neck and scalp arteries. The dilation of these arteries triggers the release of pain-producing substances called prostaglandins from various tissues and blood cells. Chemicals that cause inflammation and swelling and substances that increase sensitivity to pain are also released. The circulation of these chemicals and the dilation of the scalp arteries stimulate the pain-sensitive nerve endings called nociceptors. The result, according to this theory, is a throbbing pain in the head.

Migraine attacks commonly take one of two forms. The most common is called migraine without aura (common migraine), accounting for 85 percent of all migraine headaches. These are characterized by episodes of severe, often throbbing pain that may affect only one side of the head, although both sides may be affected. The signature of these headaches is that they are usually, but not always, associated with a feeling of being sick to the stomach or of sensitivity to light, sound, or movement of the body. Typically the sufferer wishes to lie down in a dark and quiet room and wait for the storm to pass. Often, those people close to a patient can predict when headache will occur because of changes in the patient's behavior, which may range from depression to exhilaration. If the headache is not relieved early by sleeping it off, it may wax and wane for days, accompanied by appetite loss, nausea, or vomiting—hallmarks of the so-called sick headache.

The second most common type is called migraine with aura (classical migraine). The aura of this type of headache, which accounts for most of the remaining 15 percent of migraines, is caused by a disturbance in the nervous system that precedes the headache. Typical disturbances would involve bright flashing lights, black spots, a partial loss of vision, or a feeling of pins and needles moving over one limb or one side of the body. These disturbances are usually short-lived, less than one hour for most sufferers, and almost invariably disappear, leaving no long-lasting effects.

OTHER VASCULAR HEADACHES

Toxic headache

After migraine, the most common type of vascular headache is the so-called "toxic" headache experienced during a fever. Pneumonia, flu, measles, mumps, and tonsillitis are examples of the diseases that can cause severe toxic vascular headaches.

Chemical headache

Repeated exposure to nitrite compounds can result in a dull, pounding headache that may be accompanied by a flushed face. Nitrite, which dilates blood vessels, is found in such diverse products as heart medicine and dynamite. Hot dogs and other meats containing sodium nitrite can also cause headaches. Headaches can also result from exposure to other poisons, even common household products like insecticides, carbon tetrachloride, and lead. Children who eat flakes of lead paint may develop headaches. So may anyone who has contact with lead batteries or lead-glazed pottery. Painters, print-makers, and other artists may experience headache after exposure to art materials that contain chemicals called solvents. Solvents, like benzene, are found in turpentine, spray adhesives, rubber cement, and inks.

"Chinese restaurant headache"

This can occur when a susceptible person eats foods prepared with monosodium glutamate (MSG). Soy sauce, meat tenderizer, and a variety of packaged foods might contain this chemical, which is used as a flavor-enhancer.

Hangover headache

Jokes are often made about alcohol hangovers, but the headache associated with "the morning after" is no laughing matter. The hangover headache may be reduced by taking honey, which speeds alcohol metabolism, or caffeine, a constrictor of dilated arteries. Caffeine, however, can cause headaches as well as cure them. Heavy coffee drinkers often get headaches when they try to break the caffeine habit.

External compression headache
This refers to the occasional complaint of steady headache provoked by a tight hat or band on the head.

"Ice-cream headache"
Such headaches develop in cold weather, after a swim in cold water, or after the ingestion of cold food.

Benign cough headache
If a patient suffers head pain brought on by coughing over a long period of time, intercranial pathology should be ruled out as a cause. This syndrome may develop in midlife or later, last several months, and spontaneously resolve.

Benign exertional headache
These may be brought on by exercise of any sort; like the external compression headache, they are more common in those who suffer from migraine. If these headaches continue to interfere with athletic endeavors, they may be prevented by specific therapy for migraine.

Headache associated with sexual activity
These usually start as a dull diffuse pain and intensify as sexual excitement increases, sometimes becoming very intense at the time of orgasm. Occasionally, patients complain of "postcoital headache" that is intensified when they are upright but is relieved when they recline.

Drug-induced headache
Headaches are one of the most common side effects to prescription and over-the-counter drugs, making it very diffi-

---

DRUGS THAT MAY CAUSE HEADACHES

Amyl nitrate
Bromocriptine (Parlodel)
Caffeine
Clinidine (Catapres)
Ergotamine (Ergostat)
Etretinate
Hydralazine (Alazines)
Ibuprofen (Advil)
Indomenthacin (Indocin)
Labetalol (Normodyn)
Naproxen (Naprosyn)
Nifedipine (Procardia)

Nitrofurantoin (Macrodantin)
Nitroglycerin
Perhexilene (Pexid)
Phenytoin sodium (Dilantin)
Propranolol (Inderol)
Sulindac (Clinoril)
Terbutaline (Brethine)
Tetracyclines
Theophylline (Theophyl)
Tolmetin (Tolectin)
Trimethoprim/sulfamethoxazole
Warfarin (Coumadin)

DRUGS THAT MAY WORSEN PREEXISTING HEADACHES

Estrogen administered cyclically
Danazol (Danocrine)
Progesterone (Progelan)

---

cult to list all potential problem medicines. However, those listed above can cause significant headaches.

Sinus Headaches

In a condition called *acute sinusitis*, a viral or bacterial infection of the upper respiratory tract spreads to the membrane that lines the sinus cavities. When one or all four of these cavities are filled with bacterial or viral fluid, they become inflamed, causing pain and sometimes headache. The particular cavity affected determines the location of the sinus headache. Chronic sinusitis may be caused by an allergy to such irritants as dust, ragweed, animal hair, and smoke.

The sinuses are bony cavities behind, above, and at each side of the nose and opening into the nasal cavity. They act as a sound box to give resonance to the voice. Like the nasal passages, the sinuses are lined with mucous membranes, which react to infection by producing mucus. This incapacitates infecting bacteria. Because the openings from the nose into the sinuses are very narrow, they quickly become blocked when the mucous membrane of the nose becomes swollen during a cold, hay fever, or catarrh, and then the infection is trapped inside the sinus. Chronic sinusitis may occur if one or more of the drainage passages from the sinuses to the nose becomes blocked. This can cause a dull pain across the face, in the temples, around the eyes, and in the head.

The herbal approach to these problems can be both indirect and direct. The indirect approach regards upper respiratory disease within the context of the person's health. Sometimes, the overproduction of mucus is an attempt by the body to discharge waste material that is not being properly eliminated by the bowels, the kidneys, and the skin. In such cases, the herbalist may prescribe bitter tonics such as gentian to encourage regular bowel movements; diuretic herbs such as dandelion leaf, which encourages kidney elimination of retained fluids and waste materials; or diaphoretic herbs such as yarrow or boneset, which stimulate skin elimination.

A direct approach would involve using actively analgesic herbs to kill the pain. There are a number of very effective plants that can do this, but they are unfortunately unavailable for general use. It is these very plants that were the original source of the prescription painkillers. The problem with these herbs as well as with the drugs is one of potential dependency.

A diet that reduces mucus production is also essential. In particular, a fruit fast for two or three days can help clear a system clogged and overburdened by toxic wastes. Hot lemon drinks reduce mucus production and so do garlic, onions, and horseradish (grate the fresh root into cider vinegar or lemon juice and eat a little each day). Mustard and aromatic herbs like oregano may also be added to food. Extra zinc and vitamin C will help build up the body's resistance to infection.

Sometimes emotional factors like suppressed grief can lead to blocked upper respiratory passages. In these cases, a good cry can free this blocked energy and alleviate the problem. Some cases of chronic mucus production are due to allergy.

The herbal approach to sinus headaches is to clear the sinuses rather than simply to kill the pain. Antimicrobal herbs are pivotal in the treatment of this often entrenched condition. These herbs will help the body deal with any infection present and also support the immune system in resisting the development of secondary infection. Remedies known as anticatarrhals will ease the symptomatic discomfort that is characteristic of this problem, also helping the body in the removal of the buildup of mucus in the sinus cavities.

Sinus Headache Formula

- Echinacea
- Elder flowers
- Goldenrod
- Wild indigo

Combine equal parts of the tinctures of these herbs and take ½ teaspoon of the combination three times a day.

A steam inhalant is also an effective technique for treating upper respiratory catarrh and sinusitis. In a bottle, mix 2 tablespoons of compound tincture of benzoin with ½ teaspoon eucalyptus oil, 6 drops peppermint oil, 5 drops lavender oil, and 5 drops pine oil. Shake well. Put a teaspoonful of this mixture in a bowl with 1 pint boiled water. Cover the head and the bowl with a towel or cloth and inhale. Be sure to keep your eyes closed to avoid irritation.

Certain foods, especially dairy products and wheat, seem to predispose people toward sinusitis because they provoke excessive formation of mucus. During an acute attack of sinusitis, all dairy and wheat-based foods must be excluded for several days, and people who have chronic or repeated attacks are advised to exclude these foods completely for several months, reintroducing them in very small amounts, if at all. Goat's and sheep's milk products are sometimes better tolerated than cow's milk. Acupuncture is a very effective therapy for sinusitis and can be used along with herbal therapy.

2

Green Medicine for Relieving Headaches

There is an abundance of plants that might be considered "headache" herbs. Unfortunately, they don't always work for all people! A representative listing would include the following commonly available remedies:

Chamomile	Peppermint
Dandelion root	Pulsatilla
Elder flower	Rosemary
Feverfew	Rue
Ginger	Skullcap
Lavender	Thyme
Lemon balm	Valerian
Marjoram	Wood betony

None of these plants are painkillers in the strict sense, that is, they do not block the experience of pain. An example of a medicinal plant that does block pain is the opium poppy. The most effective plant painkillers are controlled by law as they can potentially lead to dependency and addiction. Because of that, it is often more effective in practice to use indirect pathways. The herbs listed here appear to work by addressing the cause of the pain rather than the experience of pain. Being anti-inflammatory and muscle-relaxing antispasmodic herbs, they alleviate the processes that underlie most muscle contraction and tension headaches.

"Natural Aspirin"

A large range of plants contain natural "aspirin-type" chemicals called salicylates. It is worth noting that the whole aspirin group of drugs was originally isolated from plant sources. In fact, the name *aspirin* comes from the old botanical genus name for meadowsweet, *Spirea aspirin*, and salicylate derives from willow's Latin name, *salix*. Those herbs with significant quantities of salicylates have a marked anti-inflammatory effect, without the dangers to the stomach of aspirin itself. In fact, meadowsweet, rich in salicylates, can be used to staunch mild stomach hemorrhage even though pharmaceutical salicylates can cause such problems. Other plants rich in such constituents include willow bark, wintergreen, birch, many of the poplars, and black haw.

Salicylates are indeed "aspirinlike" in terms of their chemistry, but their properties are subtly different. The main difference is that salicylates do not cross what is known as the blood-brain barrier and so cannot directly affect neurons or block pain transmission. No other body organ is so absolutely dependent on a constant internal environment as is the brain. Other body tissues can withstand the rather small fluctuations in the concentrations of hormones, ions, and nutrients that continually occur, particularly after eating or exercising. If the brain were exposed to such chemical changes, uncontrolled neuron activity might result.

Consequently, neurons are kept separated from blood-borne substances by a so-called blood-brain barrier composed of the least permeable capillaries in the whole body. Only water, glucose, some amino acids, and respiratory gases pass easily through the walls of these capillaries.

In practice, then, herbs rich in this group of constituents are most useful in inflammations of muscles, bones, and connective tissue caused by conditions such as osteoarthritis or sports injuries. Thus, they are of great help in headaches that stem from such causes and are far less helpful in stress or tension headaches.

The analgesic and fever-lowering actions of salicylates are believed to be due to their ability to interfere with the transmission of signals to parts of the hypothalamus, leading to an increase in peripheral blood flow and sweating. Salicylates are also believed to suppress the synthesis of inflammatory prostaglandins, influence arachidonic acid metabolism, increase corticoid levels, and inhibit hyaluronidase, thereby reducing inflammation.

Unlike aspirin, willow preparations do not inhibit cyclooxygenase in thrombocytes or the aggregation of platelets, suggesting a different mechanism of action than those associated with salicylates. Because of this, willows and other salicin-containing herbs should not be used as substitutes for aspirin as a preventive protocol against strokes and heart attacks.

Essential Oils and Aromatherapy

Aromatherapy, a healing system based on the external application of the essential oils found in aromatic herbs, has much to offer in the relief of headaches. Particularly effective oils are lavender, rosemary, marjoram, chamomile, and peppermint, either separately or in combination.

Lavender can be rubbed on the temples or made into a cold compress and applied to the temples, forehead, or the back of the neck. Equal parts of lavender and peppermint may be even more effective, for lavender has the ability to enhance the action of other oils when it is used in blends.

If the headache is caused by catarrh or sinus infection, inhalations with lavender, peppermint, rosemary, or eucalyptus will usually be very effective in both relieving the headache and clearing the congestion causing it. All these oils are antiseptic and will combat the nasal infection and give immediate relief of symptoms.

The following descriptions include oils that are not specific for headaches but will be found useful in certain causes of headaches. The best way to use this list is to first have an insight into the cause of a specific headache; for example, is it related to stress, worry, food sensitivities, etc.? On this basis, the relevant essential oil can then be identified to address the cause rather than the result.

Essential Oil	Properties
Bergamot	Antidepressant, antiparasitic, anti-inflammatory, antiseptic. Enhances immunity; treats genital, urinary, mouth, and throat infections, flu, herpes, shingles and chicken pox; aids digestion. It is a traditional Italian folk medicine for fever and intestinal worms.
Chamomile	Anti-inflammatory, antiallergenic, digestive, relaxant, antidepressant. Used to treat the inflammation of sore muscles, sprains, tendons, and joints as well as headaches,

Essential Oil	Properties
CHAMOMILE *cont'd.*	diarrhea, digestive tract ulcers, asthma, and allergies. It helps reduce indigestion, PMS, menstrual pain, liver damage, and children's hyperactivity. It also destroys various types of intestinal worms and improves immune system activity.
CLARY SAGE	Antidepressant, relaxant, eases muscle and nervous tension, pain, menstrual cramps, PMS, and menopause problems such as hot flashes. It also stimulates adrenals and is a European remedy for sore throat. Used to treat postpartum depression and stress-related conditions.
CYPRESS	Astringent, stimulating to circulation, antiseptic. Treats low blood pressure, poor circulation, varicose veins, and hemorrhoids. It alleviates laryngitis, spasmodic coughing, lung congestion, urinary problems, and cellulite. It is a deodorant and reduces excessive fluids in the body associated with conditions such as diarrhea and runny nose.
EUCALYPTUS	Decongestant, antiviral, antibacterial, stimulant. Treats sinus and throat infections, fever, flu, chicken pox, and herpes. It is specific for thin mucus with chills and lack of thirst.
GERANIUM	Balancing to mind and body, antifungal, anti-inflammatory. A light adrenal stimulant and hormonal normalizer; treats PMS, menopause, fluid retention, breast engorgement, and sterility.

Continued

Essential Oil	Properties
HELICHRYSUM	Antidepressant, treats infection and inflammation of chronic cough, bronchitis, fever, muscle pain, arthritis, phlebitis, and liver problems, and counters allergic reactions such as asthma. Used to lift depression, lethargy, nervous exhaustion, and stress.
LAVENDER	Excellent first-aid oil; antiviral, antibacterial, boosts immunity, antidepressant, anti-inflammatory, antispasmodic. Used to treat lung, sinus, and vaginal infections, including *candida*. An excellent treatment for laryngitis and asthma. It relieves muscle pain, headaches, insect bites, cystitis, and other inflammation. It also treats digestive disturbances, including colic.
MARJORAM	Antispasmodic, anti-inflammatory, antiseptic. A strong sedative, eases muscle spasms, tics, menstrual cramps, headaches (especially migraines), and stiff joints. Treats spasmodic coughs, colds, flu, laryngitis, and hypertension and is a light laxative. Also helps normalize blood pressure.
NEROLI	Antidepressant, aphrodisiac. Neroli treats diarrhea and circulation problems such as hemorrhoids and high blood pressure. Used to counter emotional shock, mental confusion, nervous strain, anxiety, fear, and lack of confidence.
PEPPERMINT	Digestive; clears sinuses, antiseptic, decongestant, stimulant. Peppermint alleviates digestive tract spasms, indigestion, nausea,

Essential Oil	Properties
PEPPERMINT *cont'd.*	ulcers, irritable bowel syndrome, and helps destroy bacteria, viruses, and parasites in the digestive tract. It also clears sinus and lung congestion and is used to treat muscle spasms and inflammation.
ROSEMARY	Stimulating to circulation, relieves pain, decongestant, improves circulation. One of the best stimulants, it also lowers cholesterol, eases muscle and rheumatism pains, and treats lung congestion, sore throat, and canker sores. It stimulates the nervous system, motor nerves, adrenals, and a sluggish gallbladder. It is often used in penetrating liniments.
TEA TREE	Antifungal, antiyeast, antibacterial. A good immune system tonic that fights lung, genital, urinary, vaginal, sinus, and mouth infections. It counters fungal infections and viral infections such as herpes, shingles, chicken pox, *candida*, thrush, and flu.
YLANG-YLANG	Strong sedative, antispasmodic. Helps to lower blood pressure, tempers depression, fear, and anger; aphrodisiac in small doses. High concentration can produce headaches or nausea.

Essential oils can have an impact not only on physical issues such as muscle tension and inflammation but also on emotional states. The following summary of the psychological indications for the essentials oils comes from an excellent and comprehensive guide entitled *Aromatherapy* by Kathi Keville and Mindy Green.

Emotion	Oils
ANGER	Basil, Chamomile, Cinnamon, Coriander, Frankincense, Geranium, Hyssop, Jasmine, Lavender, Melissa, Neroli, Pine, Rose, Rosewood, Ylang-ylang.
ANXIETY	Basil, Benzoin, Bergamot, Camphor, Cardamom, Chamomile, Cypress, Fennel, Frankincense, Geranium, Jasmine, Juniper, Lavender, Marjoram, Melissa, Nutmeg, Patchouli, Peppermint, Petitgrain, Pine, Rose, Rosemary, Rosewood, Sandalwood, Ylang-ylang.
APATHY	Geranium, Jasmine, Neroli, Patchouli, Peppermint, Pine, Rose, Rosemary, Rosewood, Sage.
CONFUSION	Basil, Camphor, Cardamom, Cedar, Cinnamon, Cypress, Frankincense, Helichrysum, Hyssop, Jasmine, Lavender, Lemon, Marjoram, Neroli, Patchouli, Peppermint, Sandalwood.
DEPRESSION	Basil, Bergamot, Chamomile, Clary sage, Coriander, Frankincense, Geranium, Helichrysum, Lavender, Lemon neroli, Patchouli, Peppermint, Petitgrain, Pine, Rose, Rosewood, Sandalwood, Vetivert, Ylang-ylang.
FEAR	Basil, Chamomile, Coriander, Fennel, Hyssop, Jasmine, Melissa, Neroli, Orange, Rose, Thyme.
FORGET-FULNESS	Basil, Bay, Coriander, Melissa, Rosemary, Ylang-ylang.

Emotion	Oils
GRIEF	Cypress, Hyssop, Jasmine, Marjoram, Rose, Rosemary, Sage.
HYPER-SENSITIVITY	Cedar, Chamomile, Clary sage, Eucalyptus, Geranium, Hyssop, Juniper, Lavender, Marjoram, Myrrh, Neroli, Patchouli, Rose, Ylang-ylang.
IMPATIENCE	Bergamot, Camphor, Chamomile, Fennel, Frankincense, Jasmine, Lavender, Marjoram, Myrrh, Rose.
INSOMNIA	Bergamot, Chamomile, Cypress, Frankincense, Geranium, Jasmine, Lavender, Lemon, Marjoram, Melissa, Myrrh, Neroli, Nutmeg, Patchouli, Petitgrain, Rose, Sage, Sandalwood, Ylang-ylang.
INSTABILITY	Anise, Benzoin, Bergamot, Camphor, Chamomile, Cypress, Geranium, Helichrysum, Hyssop, Lavender, Lemon, Marjoram, Myrrh, Rosemary, Sandalwood, Thyme.
IRRITABILITY	Cedar, Cinnamon, Clary sage, Cypress, Melissa, Neroli, Orange, Patchouli.
MELANCHOLY	Benzoin, Frankincense, Lavender, Marjoram, Melissa, Peppermint, Rose, Rosemary, Rosewood, Sandalwood, Thyme.
PANIC/SHOCK	Bay, Camphor, Chamomile, Clary sage, Coriander, Eucalyptus, Jasmine, Lavender, Melissa, Orange, Patchouli, Petitgrain, Peppermint, Rosewood, Vetivert, Ylang-ylang.

Continued

Emotion	Oils
STRESS	Anise, Basil, Bay, Bergamot, Cardamom, Chamomile, Clary sage, Eucalyptus, Fennel, Frankincense, Helichrysum, Juniper, Lavender, Lemon, Marjoram, Neroli, Nutmeg, Orange, Peppermint, Rose, Rosewood, Sage, Sandalwood, Thyme, Ylang-ylang.

There are a range of ways to use essential oils. The dilutions given below are for adults, so halve them for children, and use them at quarter strength for infants. Be careful with essential oils, always dilute them, and *never* use them internally.

Massage oils. Always dilute oils before applying them to the skin. Use a carrier oil such as sweet almond oil, jojoba oil, or any other pure, unblended vegetable oil. Do not use mineral oil; unlike vegetable oils, they will not be absorbed by the skin. Usually 3 to 5 drops of essential oil to 2 teaspoons of a carrier oil is appropriate.

Baths. Add up to 5 drops of pure essential oil to a bath full of warm water. Float the oil on the surface and stir with your hand before relaxing in the bath for ten to fifteen minutes. For a hand or foot soak, use 2 to 3 drops in a bowl of warm water. Add 20 to 40 drops to 1 cup of bath salts.

Inhalation. Add 2 to 5 drops of essential oil to a bowl of hot water, cover your head with a towel, and inhale the fragrant steam, or put 1 to 2 drops directly onto a cotton ball for a convenient way to inhale the aroma.

Tension Headaches

Herbal medicine has the most to contribute in the alleviation of tension headaches because it helps to ease anxiety and serves as a component of stress management programs. This is discussed in depth in Part I of this book.

If a period of stress is predictably about to occur, it can be prepared for ahead of time, as herbs, diet, and lifestyle changes will minimize the impact. Nervine relaxants can be used regularly as gentle soothing remedies. Those listed below are examples. These herbs can be taken as teas or cold drinks, infused in massage oil, or used in relaxing footbaths or full baths.

Chamomile	Mugwort
Lavender	Oats
Lemon balm	Skullcap
Linden blossom	Vervain

A daily supplement of the B-complex vitamins and vitamin C is also helpful. As well as responding to stress in a healthy way by using herbs and improving the diet, you can try to soften the impact of the various stressors. It helps to reevaluate choices. Ask yourself these questions:

- Are you doing what you really want to do?
- If not, what would you rather be doing?

Give yourself permission to ask some questions about yourself and your lifestyle without censoring any of the answers that may come up. After pinpointing inner motivations, choices can be made about what you want to do about them. Relaxation exercises and an honest reevaluation of both lifestyle and life goals are invaluable.

Tension Headache Formula I

One possible prescription for stress and tension-related headaches is as follows:

- 2 parts skullcap
- 2 parts valerian
- 1 part oats

As a tincture, take ½ teaspoon of this mixture three times a day. As a tea, infuse 2 teaspoons dried mixture in a cup of boiling water for ten to fifteen minutes and drink three times a day.

Tension Headache Formula II

Stress reactions often have accompanying physical symptoms, so here is an example of one possible prescription for acute stress associated with indigestion and palpitations:

- 2 parts skullcap
- 2 parts valerian
- 1 part chamomile
- 1 part motherwort
- 1 part mugwort

As a tincture, take 1 teaspoon of this mixture three times a day. As a tea, infuse 2 teaspoons dried mixture in 1 cup boiling water for ten to fifteen minutes and drink three times a day.

Motherwort supports the relaxing of the other nervines but also has a specific calming impact upon heart palpitations.

Massage or Bath Oil Formula

In Aromatherapy, *authors Kathi Keville and Mindy Green recommend the following combinations for headache relief:*

- 3 drops lavender oil
- 2 drops clary sage oil
- 2 drops neroli
- 2 drops marjoram oil
- 2 drops ylang-ylang oil
- 1 drop chamomile oil
- 1 ounce carrier oil

Bath Oil Formula

- 3 drops chamomile oil
- 2 drops lavender oil
- 2 drops marjoram oil
- 2 drops thyme oil
- 1 drop coriander oil

Disperse the oils in a bathtub filled with warm water. Soak in the bath for twenty to thirty minutes. Repeat as necessary.

Massage Oil Formula for Neuralgia

Neuralgia, or nerve pain, is best remedied by treating the cause, although essential oils do alleviate the pain, especially when used in conjunction with massage.

- 5 drops helichrysum oil
- 3 drops chamomile oil
- 2 drops marjoram oil
- 2 drops lavender oil
- 1 ounce carrier oil

Combine ingredients and use for massage.

Chamomile Muscle-Relaxing Compresses

Hot chamomile compresses work well for the relaxation of painful tense muscles. Prepare a strong infusion with 1 full cup of chamomile flowers and 2 quarts of boiling water; cover with a lid and allow to steep for about ten minutes, then strain off through a sieve. Dip one cloth into the infusion, wring it out, and place it as hot as tolerable on the back, shoulders, and neck. Soak the other cloth in the hot infusion, wring it out, and place it on top of the first one. Now turn both cloths over so that the fresh hot compress is against the patient's skin. Remove the upper towel and soak it in the mixture. Repeat the procedure ten to twenty times until there is a sense of relaxation and loss of tension.

Migraine Headaches

It would be claiming far too much to say that herbal medicine can cure migraine. However, when selected with care, certain plants have much to offer in the amelioration and control of this distressing problem. By far the most important is a common roadside plant called feverfew.

Feverfew (*Tanacetum parthenium*) is commonly used in European herbal medicine as a specific remedy for the treatment of migraine. It is also the best example of a remedy long known to medical herbalists that has also recently been accepted and used by allopathic medicine. It has been used throughout recorded medical history as a bitter tonic and remedy for severe headaches. Through wide media coverage in recent years, the herb has gained a well-deserved reputation as a "cure" for migraine. Clinicians at the London Migraine Clinic observed that patients were reporting marked improvements when they took the herb. Thankfully, these doctors had the inquiring and open minds of true scientists and so started their own investigations into the claims for feverfew. Clinical observations were soon reported in peer-reviewed medical journals.

The first double-blind study was done at the London Migraine Clinic, using patients who reported being helped by feverfew. Seventeen patients who regularly ate fresh leaves of feverfew daily to prevent migraine were invited to participate in a double-blind, placebo-controlled trial of the herb. Of these, eight patients received capsules containing freeze-dried feverfew powder, and nine received a placebo. Those patients who received the placebo (and as a result stopped using feverfew) had a significant increase in the frequency and severity of headaches, nausea, and vomiting during the six months of the study as well as the reemergence of untoward effects during the early months of treatment. The group given capsules of feverfew, on the other hand, showed no change in the lack of symptoms of migraine, providing clear evidence that feverfew can prevent attacks of migraine. Two patients in the placebo group who had been in complete remission during self-treatment with feverfew leaves developed a recurrence of incapacitating migraine and had to withdraw from the study. The resumption of self-treatment led to renewed remission of symptoms in both patients. This led the researchers to strongly suggest the use of feverfew for all migraine sufferers.

Another double-blind study was performed at the University of Nottingham. The results of the study clearly demonstrated that feverfew was effective in reducing the number and severity of migraine attacks and confirmed that a daily intake of feverfew prophylactically prevents attacks of migraine.

Follow-up studies to clinical results have shown feverfew works in the treatment and prevention of migraine headaches by inhibiting the release of blood vessel–dilating substances from platelets, inhibiting the production of inflammatory substances and reestablishing proper blood vessel tone.

The effectiveness of feverfew is dependent upon adequate levels of parthenolide, the active ingredient. The preparations used in the clinical trials had a parthenolide content of 0.2 percent. The dosage of feverfew used in the London Migraine Clinic study was one capsule containing 25 mg of the freeze-dried pulverized leaves twice daily. In the Nottingham study, it was one capsule containing 82 mg of dried powdered leaves once daily. While these low dosages may be effective in preventing an attack, a higher dose (1 to 2 grams) is necessary during an acute attack. Feverfew is extremely well tolerated and no serious side effects have been reported. However, chewing the leaves can result in small ulcerations in the mouth and swelling of the lips and tongue. This condition occurs in about 10 percent of users.

The venerable English herbalists Gerard and Culpepper would not have been surprised at all at these findings. It is a pity that the patients given the placebo had to go through the renewed migraine attacks to demonstrate something already well known to herbalists and the patients themselves.

Pharmacologists are putting great attention on the humble "weed," feverfew, in the search for a new class of effective and profitable antimigraine and analgesic drugs. Since the simple dried or fresh leaf of feverfew is such an excellent formulation for preventing migraine, why don't doctors prescribe it? The reasons are social, political, and economic as well as medical. Since the plant is grown by nature free of charge and is not patentable, there is no profit in it for the pharmaceutical industry. Moreover, most of the information passed on to doctors is generated by that industry.

Following the clinical clues, pharmacologists are finding active components in the plant. Part of the herb's action appears to be its ability to inhibit secretion of the granular contents from platelets and neutrophils in the blood. This may be relevant to the therapeutic value of feverfew in migraine and other conditions such as osteoarthritis.

The five main compounds that were identified as having this activity were parthenolide, 3-beta-hydroxy-parthenolide, secotanaparthenolide-A, canin, and artecanin, all of which are sesquiterpene lactones. The researchers say that it is very likely that these and other sesquiterpene lactones inhibit prostaglandins and histamine released during the inflammatory process, thereby preventing spasms of the blood vessels in the head that trigger migraine attacks. Other studies indicate that feverfew inhibits interactions of human platelets and polymorphonuclear leukocytes with collagen substrates. It has been suggested that its medicinal properties are related to the inhibition of secretory activity.

As with all such impressive research findings that isolate "active" ingredients, it is important not to lose sight of the importance of the whole plant activity. Considerable differences in the parthenolide content of feverfew have been observed in plants from different geographical localities. Similarly, commercial preparations of dried feverfew usually contain varying amounts of the active principle. For this reason, standardized preparations are often used today. A daily dosage of 125 mg of a dried feverfew leaf preparation from *Tanacetum parthenium*, containing at least 0.2 percent parthenolide, is considered appropriate for the treatment and prevention of migraines. This equates to approximately 250 mcg of parthenolide daily.

Feverfew is a long-term treatment, not an immediate cure for a migraine attack. Clinical experience suggests that four to six weeks are usually required to note an initial response. However, average duration of use will vary among migraine patients. Success should be measured by decreased frequency, severity, and duration of migraine attacks. Don't use feverfew if you are pregnant or breast-feeding. If you are already taking prescription medications for migraines, consult a healthcare professional before using feverfew.

Some people find that regular use of feverfew is enough to control or even clear their migraines. However, for others, additional herbal support may also be in order. Ginkgo offers some very relevant properties mainly due to its ability to tone the blood vessel walls as well as reduce the tendency for platelet clumping to occur. Ginkgo extract standardized to

24 percent flavone glycosides is recommended at a dose of 120 mg daily in two to three divided doses.

Migraine Triggers and Contributing Factors

Early signs of a headache and whatever sets it off are critical to notice. These signs may be actual beginnings of the headache or physical events that almost invariably lead to a headache. Catching the very early signs of a headache, perhaps even before pain begins but certainly before it becomes severe, can give you important clues to controlling a headache. These early signs may be symptoms of aura, aching muscles, cold hands, a general sense of tension, or any number of other indications.

A trigger for headache pain may be almost anything in one's lifestyle or environment. Triggers don't cause the pain; rather, they activate an already existing chemical mechanism

---

Mrs. Gosling's Formula for Migraine

Many phytotherapists in Britain focus upon supporting the liver in migraine treatments. As an example, consider the following mixture suggested by Nalda Gosling, F.N.I.M.H., one of Britain's most respected herbal clinicians.

Mix equal parts of the following dried herbs:

- Motherwort
- Vervain
- Dandelion root
- Centaury
- Wild carrot

Simmer ¾ ounce of this mixture for fifteen minutes in 2 cups of water. Strain. Drink 4 to 6 ounces of this tea three times a day.

European Folk Remedy for Migraine

Make a tea mixture of the following dried herbs:

- 2 parts rosemary
- 2 parts peppermint
- 2 parts lemon balm
- 1 part sweet violet
- 1 part feverfew

Steep 1 teaspoon of this mixture in 1 cup of boiling water for ten to fifteen minutes. Strain and drink three times a day.

This tea has a very fine flavor and can be enjoyed daily. Homeopathy and traditional herbalism agree that sweet violet, which hides from the sun and loves the shade, can be of help to migraine patients who cannot tolerate bright sunlight and seek darkness and shade.

Cooling Compress for Migraine

- 1 quart ice-cold water
- 2 drops peppermint oil
- 1 drop ginger oil
- 1 drop marjoram oil

Pour the water into a 2-quart glass bowl and add the essential oils. Soak a clean cloth in the water and apply it to your head, forehead, or neck at the first sign of a developing migraine. Avoid letting the compress come into contact with your eyes. Apply an ice pack over the compress to keep it cold.

in the brain. For example, does drinking red wine lead to a headache within a few hours? If so, we could call red wine a trigger.

Most people's headaches are triggered not by one factor but by the interaction of several. In general, the more triggers present at any given time, the more likely a headache is to follow. In one study, migraine patients reported an average of five triggers. This has important ramifications as it demands that triggers be observed systematically over time and that all be considered.

Factors that increase one's vulnerability to headache, but do not immediately lead to one, are called contributing or contextual factors. Such factors create a context in which a headache is more likely to be set off by triggers. Some people can develop migraine not only during a period of stress but also afterward, when their vascular systems are still reacting. Migraines that wake people in the middle of the night are also believed to result from a delayed reaction to stress.

General "toxicity," that is, any tendency to constipation, liver problems, or general congestion will be a marked trigger in some individuals. Structural, cranial, and spinal misalignments may also be involved, as may poor posture, even when not associated with overt skeletal problems.

Common headache triggers include:

- **Stress.** Particularly for chronic tension headaches or migraine, stress can be a powerful trigger. Stress can come from major life events such as a divorce or moving, but everyday hassles like commuting or a demanding boss can have an even bigger effect.

- **Emotions.** Common negative emotions such as depression, anxiety, a sense of letdown, and frustration as well as positive pleasant excitement can trigger headaches.

- **Muscle tension.** Almost all individuals with chronic headache have some degree of muscle irritation at the upper back, neck, and face. The muscle irritation is most often associated with chronic but subtle muscle tension—nothing very dramatic but going on regularly day after day. This is true for both migraine and tension-type headaches. Muscle irritation should be considered a trigger of headache pain. The type of pain triggered reflects a variety of factors, not the least of which is the type of headache to which an individual is prone. Muscle irritation can produce local pain or pain around the site of the muscle irritation, or it can refer pain to sites away from the irritated muscle. For example, muscle irritation at the back of the neck may be felt as severe pain at the temple on the same side of the head. This is called referred pain.

Chronic muscle tension may arise from a variety of causes—regular poor posture, repeated muscle strain or overuse, tightening up under stress, mannerisms such as frowning or grinding the teeth, or even bracing against headache pain itself. Eventually, this tension may lead to very tender muscles, aching with normal movement, stiffness from being in one position for a long time, pain when lying in bed for a prolonged period, or even restriction in the mobility of the neck or jaw.

- **Diet.** Between 8 and 25 percent of people with migraine can point to a particular food as a source of their attacks.
- **Change in the weather, seasons, altitude, or time zones.**
- **Change in sleep patterns and meal times.** Both too little or too much sleep can act as triggers.
- **Hormone levels.** The normal fluctuations in hormone levels during the menstrual cycle or pregnancy, or from estrogen replacement therapy, can be potent triggers. Oral contraceptives also can worsen migraine.
- **Sensory irritants,** such as glaring or flickering lights or unusual odors.

- **Polluted air or stuffy rooms.**
- **Smoking.** Suffering from chronic headache is one more good reason to quit smoking. Smoking seems to be a negative factor for those with chronic pain conditions in general. The way in which smoking tobacco might be associated with exacerbation of pain conditions is not known with certainty, but there are many possible routes, and none of them is good for the health. Smoking can cause headaches as nicotine constricts the blood vessels while inhaled carbon monoxide overly expands them, thus creating a condition that often triggers migraines and cluster headaches.
- **Blood clotting.** Another cause of headaches is blood clotting, also known as platelet aggregation. Clotting creates constriction of the arteries, which results in inadequate blood supply to the brain. This is then followed by a rebound dilation of the blood vessels, leading to headaches.

Women and Migraine

Migraine is more common in adult women than in men. Both sexes may develop migraine in infancy, but most often the disorder begins between the ages of five and thirty-five. The relationship between female sex hormones and migraine is unclear, but the association of migraine with menstrual flow seems to arise from the fluctuations in hormonal levels, especially estrogen, rather than from too much or too little of any particular hormone. Some women suffer from "menstrual migraine" around the time of their menstrual period, but the headaches may disappear during pregnancy. Many women trace the onset of their severe headaches to puberty while others develop migraine for the first time when they are pregnant. Still others are first affected after menopause.

The effect of oral contraceptives on headaches is perplexing. Some migrainous women who take birth control pills experience more frequent and severe attacks. However, a small percentage of women have fewer and less severe migraine headaches when they take birth control pills. Women who normally do not suffer from headaches may develop migraines as a side effect when they use oral contraceptives.

The choice of herbs goes beyond the use of feverfew here as the underlying hormonal issues need to be addressed. Remedies that facilitate hormone balancing should always be included, with chasteberry, also called vitex, the most directly relevant.

The first mixture for menstrually related migraine diminishes the symptoms of PMS, thus easing this headache trigger, while the second is the core treatment to be used on a daily basis.

The dosage of Formula #1 may be increased until the desired relief is experienced. The dosage regime may be

---

Hormonal Migraine Formula #1

- 2 parts skullcap
- 1 part valerian
- 1 part dandelion

Mix the tinctures together. Take 1 teaspoon as needed to alleviate symptoms.

Hormonal Migraine Formula #2

- 2 parts vitex
- 1 part feverfew

Mix the tinctures together. Take 1 teaspoon once a day through the month.

Deb Soule's Migraine Formula

Be as kind and patient with yourself as possible. Migraines usually take a few months or even longer to decrease in severity. The following herbs help to ease a migraine headache. Take as tea or tincture whenever you feel a migraine or regular headache coming on.

- 3 parts feverfew
- 2 parts ginkgo leaf
- 1 part lemon balm
- 1 part rosemary
- 1 part basil
- ½ part passionflower

Dose and use: *Pour 1 quart of hot steaming water over 6 tablespoons of herbs and steep, covered, five to fifteen minutes. Drink ½ cup every hour until symptoms subside. The herbs can also be taken as a tincture, four to six times a day, 3 to 60 drops each time.*

Diana DeLuca's Hormone Balancing Formula

A safe and effective tea that can achieve dramatic results in balancing female hormonal swings if used regularly is this mixture formulated by California herbalist Diana DeLuca:

- 3 parts vitex berries, crushed
- 1 part ginger root
- 1 part licorice root
- 1 part red raspberry leaf
- 1 part dandelion root

Make a decoction from this mixture (see page 192) and drink daily.

altered as necessary, varying time of day and quantity of dose to suit individual needs. For example, one may take the whole dose first thing in the morning or take smaller amounts at frequent intervals throughout the day.

Herbalists have developed many approaches to migraine, reflecting the diversity of people and their response to herbs.

Menopausal Formula

In European herbalism, vitex and St. John's wort are used extensively for easing the symptomatic discomfort that may accompany the menopausal transition. St. John's wort has a role in lessening any depression that might occur. Both herbs will combine well with feverfew to gradually alleviate menopausal symptoms.

- Vitex   ▪ St. John's wort

Mix equal parts of these tinctures. Take ½ teaspoon of the combination three times a day.

On page 40 is an example from a modern woman herbalist, Deb Soule, author of *The Role of Healing*.

If headaches occur frequently during menopause, along with other typical symptoms, try a tea blend of equal parts of St. John's wort, balm, skullcap, and passionflower.

3

Foods That Can Trigger Headaches

Foods precipitate migraine attacks in many people, not only due to allergies, but also because these foods contain compounds known as "vasoactive amines," which can trigger migraines by causing blood vessels to expand. Many migraine sufferers have been found to have significantly lower levels of a platelet enzyme that normally breaks down these natural dietary components. Since red wine contains substances that are potent inhibitors of this enzyme, it often triggers migraines in these individuals, especially if consumed along with high vasoactive-amine foods like cheese. Alcohol, especially red wine and beer, are among the most likely alcoholic beverages to cause problems. Congeners, the substances that give alcohol its distinguishing characteristics, may trigger migraines along with the alcohol itself.

The naturally occurring amino acid, tyramine, found in foods such as aged cheeses, Chianti wine, and pickled herring, affects several mechanisms known to be involved with migraine. Chocolate may be another trigger. But it's not clear whether chocolate causes migraine or whether a sudden craving for chocolate is caused by an impending migraine.

Caffeine can cause headaches by increasing the body's craving for it. When blood levels of caffeine drop, symptoms of withdrawal, including headache, may set in. That's why heavy coffee drinkers experience "morning headache" until they have that first cup of coffee. Headaches related to caffeine involve a dull, throbbing pain on both sides of the head and are generally not as intense as migraine headaches. Once the body rids itself of the caffeine's effects, the headaches will disappear on their own. People who suffer from caffeine headaches are often unaware of the cause, however, and so they do not avoid caffeine, causing the headaches to recur. Food additives, such as sodium nitrite in hot dogs and luncheon meats, or monosodium glutamate in many processed foods, may also trigger migraine in some people.

The following foods are known to commonly trigger headaches in sensitive people:

- Red or white wine
- Other alcoholic beverages
- Refined sugar products, e.g., sodas and candy
- Dried fruit
- Artificial additives, colorings, and preservatives, e.g., aspartame (NutraSweet)
- Nuts
- Onions
- Herring
- Chocolate
- Peanut butter
- Chicken livers

- Dairy products, especially sour cream and yogurt
- Vinegar (except white vinegar)
- Bananas (no more than half a banana per day may be tolerated)
- Anything that is fermented, pickled, or marinated
- Pods of broad beans (lima, navy, pinto, garbanzo, and peas)
- Any foods containing a large amount of monosodium glutamate (MSG)
- Caffeine: tea, coffee, and cola beverages
- Citrus fruit (one serving per day may be tolerated)
- Processed meats such as bologna, salami, sausage, pepperoni, hot dogs, and ham
- Hot fresh breads, raised coffee cakes, and raised doughnuts (may be tolerated if cool)
- Ripened cheeses such as cheddar, Emmenthaler, Gruyère, Stilton, Brie, and Camembert

General Dietary Guidelines

- Eat smaller and more frequent meals.
- Reduce fat intake.
- Reduce caffeine (coffee, tea, cola, chocolate).
- Reduce salt.
- Increase complex carbohydrates, such as peas, rice, squash, beans, corn, potatoes.
- Increase potassium-rich foods such as potatoes, asparagus, celery, apricots, grapes, carrots, broccoli, brussels sprouts, cauliflower, noncitrus fruits.

- Increase magnesium-rich foods such as dark green vegetables, legumes, whole grains.
- Limit alcohol intake.
- Limit sweets.

Consider taking the following supplements:

- Magnesium—200 to 300 mg twice daily.
- MaxEPA (fish oil)—3 to 4 grams daily with meals.

4

Other Helpful Treatments

Despite taking preventive measures, almost everyone gets a headache sometime. Here are some suggestions for immediate headache relief. Ice packs are among the most effective nondrug treatments. The earlier an ice pack is used to treat a headache, the better. Besides applying it to the painful area, try placing it on the back of the neck, forehead, and temples.

- **For tension headache.** Try heat or ice packs, a hot shower, and rest. Take a break from a stressful situation.
- **For migraine.** Sleep. Take a nap in a dark, quiet room. Press an ice pack to the back of your neck and apply gentle pressure to painful scalp areas.

Over the long term try these steps:

- **Control triggers.** (See pages 44 to 45.)
- **Keep a headache calendar.** This helps identify those factors that cause your headaches so you can avoid them.
- **Limit the use of pain relievers.**
- **If you smoke, quit.** Smoking may bring on either a migraine or a cluster headache and increase its intensity.

- **Manage stress.** Exercise regularly. However, if physical activity brings on a migraine, make sure you first warm up slowly.

Sometimes depression, anxiety, or other kinds of emotional problems are associated with chronic and severe headaches. In fact, headaches can be an important marker for depression. You may need to focus more on treating the entity of depression than on treating the symptom of headache. Consider individual or family counseling to help minimize the impact of emotional problems on your headaches. Counseling may also help reduce the negative effects your headaches may have on your family. You might also join a headache support group.

Self-Massage

The following self-massage can provide relief from headache pain. Sit comfortably in a chair, taking care to breathe freely through the diaphragm. Cradle the back of your neck with your hand and squeeze gently, slowly rolling your head from side to side. Release for a few moments, then again squeeze your neck, slightly increasing the pressure. Repeat squeezing and releasing twenty times. Next, using your fingertips, press into any areas in your neck and shoulders that are sore and tender, moving your arms and shoulders in a gentle, rhythmic motion. Continue this for several minutes, until your headache fades.

Doing this massage periodically throughout the day will often prevent headaches from reccurring. They can also be performed by a partner. As you seat yourself, have your partner stand behind you and follow the above instructions.

A PROGRESSIVE RELAXATION EXERCISE

The following exercise is one headache sufferers can use to learn how to relax and relieve the stress of muscle tension.

Lie down or lean back in a comfortable chair in a quiet room with subdued light. Take ten slow, deep breaths, taking a little longer to breathe out than you take to breathe in. The ideal timing is a two-second full inhalation followed by a slow, controlled four- or five-second exhalation. This starts the relaxation process.

Beginning with the feet, clench the toes tightly for a few seconds, then release. Then tighten the muscles of the leg, and relax. Repeat this process for the rest of the body: buttocks, back, abdomen, hands, arms, shoulders, neck, jaw, eyes, and finally the muscles of the face. Next, yawn several times, then squeeze the eyes open and shut, taking another ten deep breaths. Notice how much more relaxed you are. Continue breathing, allowing yourself to relax even more. Then resume your regular activities.

Hydrotherapy

Hydrotherapy is another method for treating headaches without drugs. Hot baths, saunas, heat lamps, and steam baths all reduce tension by increasing blood circulation. A migraine headache, for instance, can sometimes be stopped with the combination of a hot shower followed quickly by an ice-cold one. Hot water may at first increase the migraine pain by temporarily dilating blood vessels, but this paves the way for fast relief when the vessels are constricted by the cold shower.

PART II

Insomnia

5

What Is Sleep and Why Is It Important?

The *Encyclopedia Britannica* defines sleep as a "normal, easily reversible, and spontaneous state of decreased and less efficient responsiveness to external stimulation. Sleep is a regularly recurring suspension of consciousness that serves recuperative and adaptive functions. Sleep usually requires the presence of flaccid or relaxed skeletal muscles and the absence of the overt, goal-directed behavior often seen in wakeful organisms. An electroencephalogram (EEG) recording the electrical activity of the human brain shows a distinctive pattern during sleep."

This is enough to keep me awake all night!

Let me try to translate. Sleep and rest allow the body to replenish depleted energy reserves and allow us to maintain normal physical and mental functioning. Adquate sleep is essential for good physical and mental health because it is necessary for the body's restorative processes. These processes occur in harmony with the body's sleep cycles dictated by the body's natural rhythms. The cycles change into slightly more than twenty-four hours in length and are reset each day by light and other time cues. Their rhythms dictate our need for periodic rest so that sleep is as important to our biological well-being as food, water, warmth, and shelter.

Researchers have discovered that normal, restful sleep in human beings consists of four patterns of brain activity called stages. Stages 1 and 2 are considered to be "light" stages of sleep and they typically predominate in the early part of the cycle. Stages 3 and 4 are deeper, more restful periods and they tend to dominate in the latter half of sleep. All four stages come and go many times during the night. Transient awakening usually occurs during stage 1 sleep. Most dreaming occurs during stage 4, which is also know as REM (rapid eye movement) sleep.

If the normal pattern of alternating stages is disturbed, sleep may not be fully restorative. In other words, it not only matters how many hours of sleep you get, but the quality of those hours, and the sequence of sleep stages in your brain plays a role as well.

While sleeping approximately eight hours per night is vital to people's physical and mental health, dreaming is necessary for people's psychological health. Most theories of dream function state that dreams enable people to master their environments. In dreams, people integrate new experiences and solve conflicts from their waking lives. Another function of sleep and dreaming is that both assist in the processing and storage of memories.

What Happens When You Don't Get Enough Sleep?

According to a recent Gallup Poll, one in three Americans experiences occasional or frequent insomnia. Similar studies shows that 20 to 30 percent of people in other countries also suffer from sleep-related problems. Common sleep complaints reported include:

- Difficulty falling asleep
- Difficulty staying asleep
- Difficulty going back to sleep after waking up at night
- Feeling drowsy or tired on awakening in the morning
- Feeling excessively tired or sleepy during the day

Far from being a benign, harmless condition, insomnia causes thousands of deaths every year. Its total cost in terms of illness, injuries, and decreased quality of life is staggering.

Missing one night's sleep is not that bad for your body. The main effect of a poor night's sleep, or even two or three nights, is that you just get very sleepy. You also lose motivation for doing work or anything else but sleeping; it is difficult to pay attention to tasks, especially if they are boring; and your reaction time is somewhat slowed. Monotonous activities such as driving can be risky. So there are some effects, but they usually aren't critical. For most jobs, performance is not affected by one night's loss of sleep. However, making crucial judgments or doing creative thinking can be more difficult and, if a job is extremely boring, there is a decrease in performance even after the loss of just two hours of sleep on one night.

Regularly missing sleep may be a different story. After several nights without sleep, performance goes down, and you have more trouble concentrating and remembering numbers. In experiments involving sleep deprivation for long periods, it was found that a person's mood deteriorates first—joy disappears—and the person becomes very sleepy and grim. After about two or three days, most people start having minisleeps, little lapses of attention when the brain goes to slelep for only five or ten seconds and wakes right up again. By about five days, these minisleeps become longer and more numerous. By ten or eleven days, the minisleeps are so numerous and so mixed with wakefulness that you can't tell whether you are awake or asleep. You can talk and in the middle of talking have two or three slow waves of sleep. You can walk and from one step to the next you might catch a second of sleep.

Many adults get less than optimal sleep, and some have a sizable sleep debt. Like gamblers playing with borrowed money, many sleep-deprived persons live in the red of lost sleep, often compromising their responsibilities at their jobs, sometimes using drugs for temporary energy. Most employees, even in crucial jobs, are forced to keep going all day no matter how fatigued they are. What if such sleep-deprived persons are dealing with the safety of an airplane? What if they are driving a semi-truck down a crowded highway?

Sleep loss accumulates, and many people carry a dangerously large sleep debt, often unknowingly. Soon, the chronic loss of sleep can cause lapses of attention, inability to respond, slow thinking, impaired memory, erratic behavior, and irritability. Mental functions decline and judgment fades, with results serious enough to be a danger to the person as well as to society, especially when critical decisions are being made, vehicles are being driven, or dangerous machinery is being used. A person with a big sleep debt is slower to recover from stress and is much more vulnerable to infections and other illnesses. Clearly, the immune system functions considerably better after good sleep than after insomnia. A 1995 study shows that natural killer-cells (attacking foreign elements in our body) are least active in insomniacs, somewhat more active in depressed patients, and most active in normally sleeping patients. This may be one of the reasons insomniacs feel that they catch colds and other infectious diseases more frequently than is normal. Poor sleep also heightens the

effects of drinking alcohol. An insomniac's general functioning, as well as driving performance, deteriorates to a far
greater degree than that of a well-rested person who has
consumed the same amount of alcohol.

People with chronic insomnia have more than twice as
many car accidents due to falling asleep behind the wheel as
the rest of the general population. About 2 percent of those
who have no or only occasional insomnia have an accident
related to falling asleep behind the wheel, while 5 percent of
chronic insomniacs have such accidents. As the sleep debt
grows, the pressure to sleep while on the job or on the road
increases.

The consequences of insomnia range from mild daytime
drowsiness to serious injuries and even death. Accidents can
occur due to falling asleep or loss of concentration, mainly
while operating an automobile or other potentially dangerous
machinery. Many insomniacs report loss of ability to enjoy
family and social relationships. Some avoid social contact for
fear of falling asleep while visiting friends.

How Much Sleep Is Enough?

The amount of sleep needed varies tremendously between
individuals. There is no "normal" amount; different people
need different amounts of sleep. However, the amount that
any one person needs is amazingly constant. Although you
may sleep longer one night than another depending on your
circumstances, the number of hours slept over a week or a
month usually averages out very much the same; one week
usually falls within a half hour of another week. Eight hours
of sleep a night is the usual quoted average, although seven
to seven and a half hours is more accurate for most people.

Even that number is only an average and has nothing to do with what's good or bad. A good night's sleep can range from less than three hours to more than ten.

The amount of sleep that's right for you is that which enables you to feel wide awake, alert, and energetic throughout the day. In other words, the amount and quality of your sleep are usually normal if it seems so to you, and if your daytime efficiency and alertness are not decreased. The best way to determine this is by going to bed in the evening when sleepy and waking up in the morning without an alarm and noting the total time slept.

Does Sleep Change with Age?

Once a person reaches adulthood, the amount of sleep required varies only a little as you age; however, the pattern of sleep does change. The older person often sleeps more lightly, and, as the body ages, the quality of sleep usually deteriorates: sleep becomes lighter, less efficient, and less restful. The frequency of nocturnal awakenings increases (however, most people don't recall these brief awakenings). There is a gradual decrease in delta sleep, the deepest sleep, the part of sleep most associated with growth and bodily recovery. By around age fifty for men and sixty for women, there is much less of the deep delta sleep, sometimes none, so that people at these ages and older are more easily aroused by noises or other outside factors that younger people might sleep through.

Thus, the changes that occur in sleep patterns with age increase susceptibility to sleep deprivation and insomnia. There is no truth to the myth that older people sleep less during the night because they "need less sleep." They sleep less because their ability to sleep has been biologically impaired due to changes in brain functions that are beyond their direct control. Reports of insomnia tend to increase with age and are more prevalent among women, even though laboratory studies show that older men have more disrupted sleep. People who are divorced, widowed, or separated reported having insomnia more often than married people; lower socioeconomic status is also a correlate of insomnia.

What Is Insomnia?

Insomnia is insufficient, disturbed, nonrestorative sleep. This means not getting enough sleep to meet the needs of your body or to allow you to feel refreshed and energetic upon awakening and throughout the day. The National Institutes of Health define insomnia as "a disturbance or perceived disturbance of the usual sleep pattern of the individual that has troublesome consequences." These consequences may include daytime fatigue and drowsiness, irritability, anxiety, depression, and somatic complaints.

It is normal to wake up several times each night. Although most people don't recall these brief awakening episodes, insomniacs typically have trouble getting to sleep in the first place or falling back to sleep once they have awakened.

Insomnia as a concept does not apply to problems that primarily result in excessive daytime drowsiness, such as sleep apnea and narcolepsy. These disorders usually have biological causes, and while disordered nighttime sleep patterns are sometimes involved, true insomnia is an infrequent complaint.

Most people with insomnia have it on an occasional or intermittent basis. About 9 percent of the general population, however, have chronic, prolonged insomnia. Thus, at any point in time, more than 20 million Americans suffer from severe, debilitating insomnia lasting from several months to many years.

Kinds of Insomnia

Various scientific groups classify insomnia in different ways. One system divides insomniacs into people who can't fall asleep when they go to bed and people who fall asleep readily but can't stay asleep. A second system is based on how long the insomnia lasts. This system classifies insomnia as transient insomnia if it lasts just one to three nights, short-term insomnia if it lasts from four nights to three weeks, and chronic insomnia if it lasts more than three weeks. Another classification system sorts the causes of insomnia into five main categories:

1 | Insomnia associated with psychological problems

2 | Insomnia associated with medical problems

3 | Insomnia due to lifestyle

4 | Insomnia caused by poor sleep habits

5 | Primary insomnia

6

The Causes of Sleeplessness

Insomnia is a symptom that usually has a cause. Often there are multiple causes, and the ones that initiated the problem may no longer be the ones that are keeping it from resolving. When you are trying to figure out the causes of your insomnia, consider the following categories.

Medical Illness

Conditions that involve pain, shortness of breath, cough, urination, nausea, diarrhea, or other bothersome symptoms at night can often result in insomnia, such as:

- Arthritis
- Muscle aches/pains
- Lung disease/asthma
- Heart disease
- Diabetes
- Overactive thyroid
- Headaches
- Colitis

- Heartburn/reflux esophagitis
- Infections
- Hot flashes/menstrual pains
- Leg cramps
- Restless leg syndrome

Restless leg syndrome consists of abnormal sensations in both legs upon lying down. These sensations are usually described as "ants or insects crawling on my legs" and they are often relieved (temporarily) by moving the legs. The syndrome is also usually accompanied by periodic movements of both legs during sleep and is sometimes associated with diabetes, kidney disease, or circulatory problems; in the majority of cases, however, no specific cause can be found.

Psychological Illness

Any psychiatric or psychological illness can interfere with sleep. Conditions associated with increased anxiety or worry often keep people from falling asleep, whereas depressive illnesses often result in early morning awakening or trouble remaining asleep.

In addition, many prescription medications for treating psychiatric illness can also compromise sleep. Certain antidepressants, such as Prozac, Zoloft, and Paxil, can have stimulating effects. Tranquilizers such as Valium may at first help anxious people sleep, but with prolonged usage they can disturb normal sleep activity in the brain. The same is true for caffeine, nicotine, and alcohol use, which frequently increase during times of psychological stress.

Also, negative associations and other bad sleep habits that become established during periods of psychological distress can remain as lingering problems after the underlying psychological crisis has resolved. For example, poor habits such as trying too hard to get back to sleep or spending too much time lying awake in bed can become established during a period of depression and remain as causes of persistent insomnia once the depression has successfully been treated (or cleared on its own).

Biological Clock Alterations

All human beings have biological "clocks" deep within their brains. These clocks control regular fluctuations in body functions, such as hormone secretions, temperature regulation, and sleep-wake cycles. The clock controlling sleep-wake periods typically cycles every twenty-five hours (interestingly not synchronized with our twenty-four-hour day). In some people, however, this "normal" cycle can become abnormally shortened or prolonged. The commonest way this is experienced is in the form of jet lag.

Shift Work

Shift work is a common cause of sleep deprivation for millions of Americans. Working the night shift on a regular basis or working different shifts on a rotating schedule produce challenges and obstacles to maintaining a normal, healthy sleep-wake pattern. This can be especially troublesome for older individuals, since the ability to tolerate shift work (from a sleep perspective) declines significantly with age.

Medications

Prescription and OTC (over-the-counter) medicines used to treat medical or psychiatric problems can also contribute to insomnia. If you are having trouble sleeping, look very carefully at any medicines you may have been taking recently or just prior to the onset of your problem:

- Bronchodilators (asthma remedies)
- Beta blockers (used for high blood pressure, heart disease, migraines, palpitations)
- Steroids (mainly prednisone/cortisone preparations)
- Calcium blockers (used for high blood pressure, heart disease, migraines, palpitations)
- "Nondrowsy" OTC decongestants and cold remedies
- Dilantin
- Thyroid hormones

Caffeine

Caffeine is often used by people to maintain wakefulness throughout the day. Excessive use of caffeine on a daily basis, however, can lead to withdrawal symptoms including headache and sleeplessness at night. If caffeine is ingested too close to bedtime, its stimulating properties can also interfere with sleep. Caffeine is also known to cause an increase in palpitations, stomach problems, diarrhea, and restless leg syndrome in certain individuals.

Alcohol

Alcohol is commonly used by people to help them get to sleep. While this may appear to be a good thing to do, eventually it leads to further trouble. In addition to causing a dependency state, alcohol also disrupts the normal pattern of brain activity during sleep. While its sedative and calming effects help people get to sleep at first, it tends to produce increased nighttime awakenings and reduces certain types of brain activity that are needed for proper rest.

In addition to looking at any medications or insomnia-producing substances you may be currently using, also consider any medications you may have recently stopped. Sometimes disturbed sleep begins shortly after stopping a medication you've been taking for quite some time. For example, people who suddenly quit smoking often find that their sleep is disturbed. Withdrawing from alcohol, sleeping pills, or psychiatric medications can also produce temporary insomnia. Sometimes a more gradual tapering down of these agents will prevent this type of insomnia from occurring, so it is best to consult with your physician if you think this factor might be involved.

Negative Conditioning

Another common cause of insomnia is the way people respond to their inability to sleep. After not sleeping well for several days, many people become worried, frustrated, or depressed. This causes them to place added psychological pressure on themselves to sleep. This leads to increased anxiety at bedtime, which further interferes with sleep. In no time at all, a vicious cycle of "failure-worry-more failure-more worry" develops. Once established, this failure pattern becomes self-perpetuating. It can be reversed, however, by following some of the guidelines discussed in this book.

In addition, insomnia-maintaining behaviors, such as staying in bed too long when you can't sleep, can also aggravate the problem. So can performance anxiety, where the more you try to make yourself fall asleep, or the more you worry about achieving your goal, the less you are able to relax. These "secondary" causes of insomnia are very important to recognize. One good clue is that you sleep very well in places or at times that you don't normally associate with sleep. For example, you may sleep well on vacation or at a friend's home. You may have no trouble taking unplanned naps at home, while trying to sleep at bedtime is often unsuccessful.

Bad Sleep Habits

Some conditioned responses lead to bad sleep habits. These include:

- Failing to keep to a regular sleep-wake schedule
- Depriving your body of sleep by staying up to work or play on a frequent basis
- Trying to "catch up" on lost sleep during the weekend
- Watching late-night TV
- Excessive napping during the day
- Thinking of work-related problems while in bed
- Excessive time awareness or frequent clock-watching while in bed
- Feeling "too tired" to exercise during the day
- Exercising vigorously too close to bedtime
- Drinking tea or caffeine-containing colas close to bedtime

These behaviors commonly contribute to long-term insomnia. It's very important to recognize these causes, since in most instances they can be reduced or eliminated.

Recent Stressful Events

Another common cause of insomnia, particularly the short-term variety, is the occurrence of stressful events or crises in a person's life. These can include such events as:

- Loss of one's job
- Major changes affecting one's job

- Death/illness of relative or friend
- Being personally attacked or threatened
- Major life transitions (e.g., having a child, moving, getting married, graduating school)
- Developing a health or illness problem
- Financial crises
- Relationship conflicts
- Legal entanglements
- Committing a crime

In general, the successful resolution of these problems usually leads to restoration of normal sleep. However, if negative associations and bad sleep habits become established during periods of stress-induced insomnia, these secondary causes can keep one sleeping poorly.

When to Seek Medical Advice

If you are having chronic or recurring sleep problems that don't clear up with the measures discussed in this book, you should consult your healthcare provider. Also, if you are feeling severely anxious or depressed, or if your sleep is being disturbed by pain or other physical symptoms, professional help is indicated. You might need to be tested for a thyroid disorder, diabetes, or other medical problem. You might also need advice about pain medication, sleeping pills, antidepressants, muscle relaxants, or other prescription remedies.

If you are thinking about using prescription sleeping pills, you should discuss this decision with your doctor. All major sleeping pills interfere with normal brain wave patterns during sleep. All can affect daytime functions, including memory, concentration, and rapid response times. In addition, the abrupt withdrawal of sleeping medication after prolonged use can lead to "rebound" insomnia.

Sleeping pills should definitely be avoided if you are pregnant, are possibly pregnant, or are considering getting pregnant. They should also be avoided if you are elderly, if you work in a dangerous occupation, if you tend to drink alcohol, if you are taking other prescription medications, if you have severe kidney or liver disease, if you have any suicidal thoughts or tendencies, or if your bed partner complains that you snore excessively (this may be a sign of sleep apnea, which can worsen with certain sleeping pills).

You should always use the lowest dose of medication that helps you to sleep and discontinue usage as quickly as possible. Infrequent usage may sometimes be justified, but long-term dependence should generally be avoided. However, never abruptly stop any sleeping medication you've been taking for some time without first consulting with your physician.

7

Green Medicine for a Good Night's Sleep

The key to successful treatment of insomnia is to find the cause and deal with it. This may be anything in the realm of human life, from deep grief to constipation. Psychological issues often need attention, but then so do health problems causing pain or discomfort. Dietary indiscretions must be identified as must environmental factors (e.g., freeway noise or a snoring spouse). Insomnia can push the practitioner's diagnostic skills to the limit, making the orthodox physician's free and easy prescribing of sleeping medications at least understandable.

The herbal repertoires of the world abound in plants that can prove successful in the search for a good night's sleep. However, it can sometimes be helpful to think in terms of groups of herbs that share properties. These are often called the actions of the plants. Herbal actions that might be indicated for the processes involved underlying insomnia follow.

Hypnotics

Hypnotics are herbal remedies that will help to induce a deep and healing state of sleep. Herbs that help you sleep have

HYPNOTIC HERBS

California poppy	Pulsatilla
Chamomile	Skullcap
Hops	Valerian
Linden	Vervain
Motherwort	Wild lettuce
Mugwort	Wood betony
Passionflower	

modes of action that vary from mild muscle-relaxing properties through volatile oils that ease psychological tensions to remedies that contain strong alkaloids that work directly on the central nervous system and put you to sleep. Some of the most effective plant hypnotics are illegal because of their addictive potential. This includes the whole range of opium poppy derivatives. The remedies mentioned here are entirely safe and have no addictive properties. Hypnotic herbs should always be used within the context of an approach to sleep problems involving relaxation, food, and lifestyle in general.

Nervines

A nervine is a plant remedy that has a beneficial effect upon the nervous system in some way. This makes the word nervine a catchall expression. To study nervines properly, it helps to differentiate them into a number of categories. It may be superfluous to point this out, but any successful treatment of nervous system problems with herbs must involve treating the whole body, heart, and mind, not simply the signs of agitation and worry. Of course, the agitation can be reduced greatly, but the whole system must be strengthened in the face of the storm. The main nervine subdivisions are:

- **Tonics.** Oatstraw, skullcap, St. John's wort
- **Relaxants.** Skullcap, valerian, vervain
- **Stimulants.** Cola, guarana

Nervine Tonics

Perhaps the most important contribution herbal medicine can make in the whole field of neurology is in strengthening and "feeding" the nervous system. In cases of shock, stress, or nervous debility, the nervine tonics strengthen and restore the tissues directly. On the other hand, they can contribute to the healing of damaged nervous tissue, whether this is due to a pathological process or physical trauma. This invaluable group of remedies is best exemplified by oats (also referred to as oatstraw), which has neither a relaxant nor stimulant effect. Ginkgo is an important tonic for the nervous system, but appears to work via its vasodilating action on the blood vessels of the brain. This will increase oxygen availability to brain cells. Other nervine tonics that have, in addition, a relaxing effect include skullcap and St. John's wort. Of these relaxing nervine tonics, skullcap is often the most effective, particularly for problems related to stress.

NERVINE TONICS WITH A RELAXING EFFECT	
Chamomile	St. John's wort
Hyssop	Vervain
Lavender	Wood betony
Skullcap	

Nervine Relaxants

This group of nervines is most important in our times of stress and confusion, alleviating many of the accompanying symptoms.

Nervine relaxants should always be used in a broad holistic way, not simply to tranquilize. Too much tranquilizing, even that achieved through herbal medication, can in time deplete and weigh heavily on the whole nervous system.

As can be seen from the list of herbs below, many of the nervine relaxants also have other properties and can be selected to aid in related problems. This is one of the great benefits of using herbal remedies to help in stress and anxiety problems. The physical symptoms that so often accompany the ill-ease of anxiety may be treated with herbs that work on the anxiety itself.

In addition, the nervine herbs that work directly on the nervous system, the antispasmodic herbs (which affect the peripheral nerves and the muscle tissue) can have an indirect

---

NERVINE RELAXANTS

Black cohosh	Motherwort
Black haw	Mugwort
California poppy	Passionflower
Chamomile	Pulsatilla
Damiana	Red clover
Hops	Skullcap
Hyssop	St. John's wort
Jamaican dogwood	Valerian
Lavender	Vervain
Lemon balm	Wild lettuce
Linden	Wood betony
Lobelia	

See the Materia Medica *for a brief discussion of some of these herbs showing their primary use and how to prepare and take them.*

relaxing effect on the whole system. When the physical body is at ease, ease in the psyche is promoted. Many of the nervine relaxants have this antispasmodic action. The hypnotic herbs, when given in lower dosages, also have a relaxing action on the mind and body.

Individualized Herbal Formulas

Often the key to successful treatment lies in focusing upon some part or function of the body that is experiencing problems that can lead to insomnia. This must be identified, and the appropriate herbs then selected. As most medicinal plants have a range of effects, it is possible to choose remedies that are relevant to the underlying problem while also being hypnotics or nervines. These can be selected by the role they play upon the system in question and not simply according to their strength as hypnotics.

- **Circulatory system.** The mild sedatives motherwort, lime blossom, and lemon balm are helpful to the cardiovascular system.

- **Respiratory system.** All the hypnotics can help as antispasmodics in conditions such as asthma, if used at the right dose. Wild lettuce eases irritable coughs.

- **Digestive system.** The relaxing nervines and carminatives are important, especially chamomile, vervain, lemon balm, hops, and valerian. The antispasmodic herbs such as hops, Jamaican dogwood, passionflower, and valerian will help with intestinal colic.

- **Urinary system.** Hypnotics are important here when used as muscle relaxants.

- **Reproductive system.** Hypnotics are helpful as muscle relaxants, especially pulsatilla and black cohosh.

- **Muscles and bones.** All hypnotics will aid in reducing muscle tension and even the pain associated with problems in this system. They may be used internally or as lotions. Especially important are valerian and black cohosh.

- **Nervous system.** All these remedies work on the nervous system.

- **Skin.** Chamomile and cowslip are healing, but otherwise the value of hypnotics here is to ensure that the body has a good recuperative rest each night.

The many relaxing/sleeping remedies can be more precisely selected on the basis of any other actions they may have, but they may also be selected on the basis of their strength, bearing in mind the very subjective nature and individual variability of human response to these herbs. We can very roughly identify three groupings:

- **Mild.** Chamomile, lemon balm, linden, red clover
- **Medium.** Motherwort, mugwort, pulsatilla, skullcap, vervain
- **Strong.** California poppy, hops, passionflower, valerian, wild lettuce

By selecting herbs that address specific health needs that are compounding or even causing sleeping difficulties, better results are obtained than simply going for a strong hypnotic. For example, an involvement of heart palpitations would indicate motherwort. As examples of ways in which different causes or additional symptoms can be taken into account in the herbal treatment of insomnia, consider the following mixtures on pages 75 to 76.

Insomnia Formula I

- Passionflower
- Valerian

Mix equal parts of the tinctures. Take ½ teaspoon of the tincture mixture thirty minutes before bedtime.

Insomnia Due to Menstrual Cramping

- Passionflower
- Motherwort
- Valerian

Mix equal parts of the tinctures. Take ½ teaspoon of the tincture mixture thirty minutes before bedtime in addition to any appropriate daytime treatments.

Insomnia Due to Indigestion

- Passionflower
- Mugwort
- Valerian
- Lemon balm

Mix equal parts of the tinctures. Take 1 teaspoon of the tincture mixture thirty minutes before bedtime in addition to appropriate daytime treatments.
  A tea (infusion) made from chamomile, linden, or lemon balm at night would also be helpful.

Insomnia Due to High Blood Pressure or Headache

- Passionflower
- Linden
- Valerian
- Crampbark

Mix equal parts of the tinctures. Take 1 teaspoon of the tincture mixture thirty minutes before bedtime in addition to any appropriate daytime treatments.
  A tea (infusion) made from linden or chamomile at night would also be helpful.

Insomnia Due to Depression

- Passionflower
- Valerian
- St. John's wort
- Mugwort

Mix equal parts of the tinctures. Take 1 teaspoon of the tincture mixture thirty minutes before bedtime in addition to any appropriate daytime treatments.

Herbal Teas

For information about preparing teas and tinctures, see How to Prepare Herbal Medicines (pages 191 to 196). Most dried herbs and tinctures can be purchased at natural food stores or from the herbal suppliers listed in the Appendix.

Every herbalist has personal favorites when it comes to teas. If you are unable to sleep because your nervous system and mind feel overactive, the following teas can be taken every day to help calm the body and ensure a good night's sleep. Here is a small range of examples:

Sleep Tea I

- St. John's wort
- Lemon balm leaves
- Valerian root
- Cowslip flowers
- Hawthorn berries
- Passionflower
- Oatstraw
- Hops
- Lavender

Combine equal parts. Pour 1 cup of boiling water onto 1 to 2 teaspoons of the dried herb mixture and leave to infuse for ten to fifteen minutes. Drink 1 cup before going to bed.

Sleep Tea II

- 3 parts skullcap
- 2 parts passionflower
- 1 part chamomile
- 1 part spearmint
- 1 part roses

Pour 1 cup of boiling water onto 1 to 2 teaspoons of the mixture and leave to infuse for ten to fifteen minutes. Drink 1 cup before going to bed.

Sleep Tea III

- 2 parts lemon balm
- 1 part skullcap
- 1 part hops
- 1 part motherwort
- 1 part chamomile

Valerian root (include with above herbs for severe insomnia), 1 part.

Infuse 2 to 3 teaspoons of the mixture for each cup of boiling water. Valerian has a strong flavor, which some people dislike, so this combination may be easier to take in tincture form, 50 drops as needed.

Sleep Tea IV

- 2 parts oatstraw
- 2 parts lemon balm
- 2 parts linden
- 1 part skullcap
- 1 part chamomile
- 1 part lavender
- 1 part vervain

Steep 1 to 2 tablespoons of herb mixture in a cup of boiling water, covered, for five to fifteen minutes. Drink warm before bedtime.

Sleep Tea V

- 2 parts peppermint
- 1 part catnip
- 1 part chamomile
- 1 part passionflower
- 1 part lemon balm

Pour 1 cup of boiling water onto 1 to 2 teaspoons of the mixture and leave to infuse for ten to fifteen minutes. Drink 1 cup before going to bed.

Herbal Tinctures

Sleep Tincture I

- Passionflower
- Skullcap
- Kava kava

Combine equal parts of the tinctures. Take 1 teaspoon thirty minutes before bed. This mixture is good added to hot spearmint tea, with honey or maple syrup to sweeten.

Sleep Tincture II

In her excellent book The Roots of Healing, *herbalist Deb Soule recommends the following combination:*

- 2 parts valerian root
- 1 part hops
- 1 part skullcap
- 1 part motherwort
- 1 part passionflower
- 1 part St. John's wort

Take 25 to 50 drops of this tincture combination thirty minutes before bedtime and take again if you awaken in the night and want to sleep more.

Sleep Pillows

Pillows made with herbs used singly or in combination are a wonderful way to promote restful sleep as well as giving a pleasant aroma to the bedroom. They are a way to augment the teas and tinctures given above. Traditionally used herbs include catnip, chamomile, hops, lavender, lemon balm, linden blossom, orange blossom, and sweet woodruff.

Make a pillowcase lining out of linen or burlap and leave open at one end. Make up a stuffing by mixing dried herbs in the following proportions:

- 2 to 3 handfuls each of peppermint, sage, and lemon balm
- 1 to 2 handfuls of lavender, dill, lemon thyme, tarragon, woodruff, red bergamot, and rosemary
- 1 to 2 tablespoons of valerian

Fill the pillow loosely with the herbs, sew closed, and put inside a pretty and soft pillowcase before use. Another possible mixture for an herbal pillow is oregano, thyme, lavender flowers, valerian root, and hop leaves. A mugwort leaf pillow is said to make for happy dreams.

Child's Sleep Pillow

Mix equal parts lavender flowers, hops, chamomile, and dill seeds. Fold a 5" x 10" piece of cloth in half, so that it measures 5" by 5" and sew the edges, leaving an opening. Combine the herbs and stuff them into the pillow; then sew the edges closed. Slip this pillow inside the child's pillowcase.

Any pillow can be augmented by using an essential oil spray such as this:

- 1 ounce distilled water
- 4 drops lavender oil
- 2 drops chamomile oil
- 2 drops orange oil
- 2 drops ylang-ylang oil

Pour the water into a spray bottle, add the essential oils, and shake to blend. Spray the mixture on your pillow and sheets or in your room before bedtime. Shake before each use.

Essential Oils and Aromatherapy

Aromatherapy, a healing system based on the external application of herbs in the form of essential oils, has much to offer those in search of restful sleep. A reliable and comprehensive guide to the safe use of these wonderful oils is *Aromatherapy* by Kathi Keville and Mindy Green, from which much of the following is taken.

A number of oils may be helpful in easing insomnia, of which the most relevant are listed below. It is very important to use them in the correct way as they are potentially toxic if taken internally. Here is a range of ways to safely use essential oils, remembering that the suggested dosages are for adults, except where indicated.

Massage Oils

Always dilute oils before applying to the skin. Use a carrier oil such as sweet almond, grapeseed, jojoba, or any other pure, unblended vegetable oil. Do not use baby oil as this is a mineral oil, and unlike vegetable oils, it will not be absorbed by the skin. Three to 5 drops of essential oil to 10 ml of a carrier oil is usually appropriate.

Baths

Add up to 5 drops of pure essential oil to a bath full of warm water. Float the oil on the surface and stir with your hand before relaxing in the bath for ten to fifteen minutes. For a hand or foot soak, use 2 to 3 drops in a bowl of warm water.

Inhalation

Add 2 drops of essential oil to a bowl of hot water, cover your head with a towel, and inhale the fragrant steam.

Insomnia during pregnancy may be safely helped with essential oils. Simply using one or two drops of lavender oil on a tissue for inhalation is often effective. Sandalwood or

ESSENTIAL OILS TRADITIONALLY USED FOR INSOMNIA

Bergamot	Mandarin
Chamomile	Marjoram
Cypress	Neroli
Frankincense	Nutmet
Geranium	Patchouli
Jasmine	Petitgrain
Lavender	Rose
Lemon balm	Sandalwood
Lemon verbena	Ylang-ylang
Linden	

ylang-ylang dropped onto nightclothes or bed linen during the whole nine months will also prove helpful.

It is interesting to note that aromatherapy is becoming widely used in hospitals in Britain, especially for sleep difficulties. Helping an elderly patient achieve a good quality, refreshing night's sleep is a bigger problem in hospitals than when the patient is at home. Lavender is the usual essential oil used to induce sleep, and a few drops of the oil on the pillow will help to induce a peaceful sleep in many patients.

Baths to Induce Sleep

Not only essential oils can be used in the bath. A pleasant way of absorbing herbal compounds through the skin is by bathing in a full body bath with 1 pint of an infusion or decoction added to the water. Any herb that can be taken internally can also be used in a bath. Herbs can, of course, also be used to give the bath an excellent fragrance.

For a bath that will bring about a deep and restful sleep,

add an infusion of one of the hypnotic herbs listed below to the bathwater. Bear in mind that although valerian and hops are very effective, their aroma is an acquired taste!

California poppy	Passionflower
Chamomile	Pulsatilla
Hops	Skullcap
Linden	Valerian
Motherwort	Wild lettuce
Mugwort	

For children with sleep problems or when babies are teething, add the following infusion to the bath:

Chamomile	Red clover
Linden	

Essential Oil Formula I

This relaxing antidepressant combination can be used as either a massage or bath oil.

- 3 drops lavender oil
- 2 drops neroli oil
- 2 drops marjoram oil
- 2 drops ylang-ylang oil
- 2 drops clary sage oil
- 1 drop chamomile oil
- 1 ounce carrier oil

Essential Oil Formula II

This blend could be used in a diffuser so that the bedroom is subtly fragranced with an aroma that facilitates sleep.

- 25 drops lavender oil
- 10 drops orange oil
- 8 drops chamomile oil
- 8 drops marjoram oil
- 6 drops ylang-ylang oil

Massage Oil for Children

This wonderfully relaxing massage oil might be used before bed to help a child sleep.

- 3 drops lavender oil
- 2 drops orange oil
- 2 ounces almond oil (or any light vegetable oil)
- 1 drop chamomile oil
- 1 drop ylang-ylang oil (optional)

Relaxing Bath Oil I

- ½ to 1 cup sea salt
- 4 drops chamomile essential oil
- 2 drops marjoram oil
- 2 drops ylang-ylang oil (optional)
- 1 drop basil oil

Add ingredients to bathtub filled with warm water and disperse well. Soak for twenty minutes.

Relaxing Bath Oil II

- 2 drops lavender essential oil
- 1 drop orange essential oil
- 1 drop chamomile essential oil
- 1 drop ylang-ylang essential oil (optional)

Add oils directly to bath when full and stir to distribute.

Instead of preparing an infusion beforehand, a handful of the herb can also be placed in a muslin bag which is suspended from the hot water tap so that the water flows through it. In this way, a very fresh infusion can be made.

Lavender water is a refreshing warm-weather splash. Keep refrigerated and dab with a cotton ball or spray on your neck and face to refresh yourself on a warm day or to relax before bedtime. To make, blend 3 cups spring water with ¼ cup vodka and 8 drops of lavender oil. Shake well before use.

Nutrition

As with all aspects of health, the food we eat (or don't eat) has a profound effect on patterns of sleep. Tryptophan, an amino acid, is a biochemical inducer of serotonin, an important neurotransmitter involved in sleep. Tryptophan is high in turkey, eggs, fish, dairy products, bananas, pineapples, whole wheat toast, and walnuts. Other dietary suggestions might include:

- Vitamin C (all tart fruits, dark leafy greens, and red peppers)
- Foods high in vitamin B complex such as brewer's yeast
- A diet rich in salads, fresh vegetables, whole grains, and fiber foods

There are also foods to avoid, either because they are stimulants to the nervous system or difficult to digest. They should be especially avoided in the afternoon and evening. Examples include meat, alcohol, hot sauces, spicy foods, coffee, and other caffeine sources. Avoid foods that are likely to cause indigestion or heartburn, such as fatty foods, heavily garlic-flavored foods (unless you are used to them), or highly spiced foods. If gas disturbs your sleep, avoid beans, cucumbers, or other foods that you have found cause gas. Many people are sensitive to monosodium glutamate (MSG). MSG can cause many symptoms, including insomnia. If you notice that insomnia occurs on nights that you have eaten Chinese food, MSG may be your problem. Some heavy salt users sleep better on less salt; others say more salt helps them sleep better.

For some people, reducing caffeine intake is easier said

than done. For others, a simple technique known as "caffeine fading" is successful. It involves reducing caffeine intake by one-half cup of coffee a day. If you are drinking more than five cups of coffee a day, you should seriously consider cutting down. The best way to proceed is to consume caffeine regularly for a week, while keeping a precise log of the times and amounts of caffeine consumed (remember that not only coffee but also chocolate, tea, cola beverages, and many headache pills contain caffeine). At the end of the week, proceed to reduce your coffee intake at the rate recommended above. Remember to have substitutes available for drinking; if you are not going to have a hot cup of coffee at your ten-minute break, you might consider having fruit juice or herbal tea, but *not* decaffeinated coffee, which still contains enough caffeine to disrupt the sleep of sensitive individuals.

It is quite common to experience some symptoms of caffeine withdrawal. When caffeine intake is reduced, the body becomes oversensitive to adenosine. In response to this oversensitivity, blood pressure drops, causing an excess of blood in the head, leading to a headache. This headache, well known among coffee drinkers, might last from one to five days, and can be eased with herbal analgesics such as willow bark or meadowsweet. It is also alleviated with caffeine intake; in fact, several analgesics contain caffeine dosages.

Often people reducing their caffeine intake become irritable, unable to work, nervous, restless, and tired, in addition to having a headache. In extreme cases, nausea and vomiting have also been reported. However, in three to five days, these symptoms vanish and a sense of well-being, heightened energy, and better sleep habits are your reward.

8

Other Ways to Relieve Insomnia

Occasional Insomnia

The best way to deal with one or two bad nights of sleep is to go to bed early the very next evening. Never make excuses for why you need to stay up late more than one or two nights in a row. Manage your schedule so you get your work done during the day, and don't treat your body like you can deprive it of sleep whenever you want.

Going to bed early is better for your body than taking a daytime nap. Napping during the day can make you less tired—and less able to sleep—at night. This can further interfere with resuming your normal sleep-wake cycle.

Short-Term Insomnia

Longer periods of insomnia, lasting one to three weeks, are often brought on by stressful life events. As already pointed out, repeated loss of sleep leads to poor daytime function and increased irritability, further decreasing ability to cope with stress, which in turn leads to more worry, anger, and frustration, which additionally compromises sleep.

If you notice you are suddenly not sleeping well for several days in a row, look for recent stressful events or conflicts in your life. When you identify them, try to resolve them quickly. Don't ignore them, put off dealing with them, or simply "hope" they will go away. Address them vigorously and successfully and your insomnia will usually resolve. Your major goal should always be to restore your previous sleep pattern just as quickly as you can. The longer insomnia lasts, the more bad habits and negative associations tend to form.

Chronic Insomnia

The best way to deal with chronic insomnia is to prevent it from becoming established in the first place. If you already have a problem that's lasted more than a month, there are some strategies most experts recommend.

Make Your Sleep Environment Safe, Quiet, and Comfortable

NOISE

Some people need absolute silence to sleep. You may be one of them, so try eliminating as much noise as possible by using carpeting, drapes, or other soundproofing, and see if that helps. If your children are the problem, get them to modify their behavior. If neighbors are the problem, see what you can do to enlist their cooperation and support. If the telephone rings late at night, try to muffle the sound, turn off the ringer, or instruct friends and relatives not to call after certain hours.

If minor noises bother you, consider using a constant background noise to help you get to sleep. Commercial devices designed to produce soothing "white noise" are also available. If these don't help, consider trying earplugs (excellent for dealing with snoring bed partners). If all else fails, soundproofing your bedroom may be in order.

DARKNESS

If you are required to sleep during the day, too much light in your sleeping environment can be a problem. If this is true for you, consider buying thicker curtains, installing window blinds, or wearing a sleep mask.

CLOCKS

Many insomniacs have an illuminated digital clock staring at them all night. When they have difficulty falling asleep, they watch it anxiously. If they wake up in the middle of the night, their first glance is toward the clock. No matter what time it is, it's always the wrong time. Other people are bothered by a loudly ticking clock.

For most people, the bedroom should be a time-free environment. Once you've decided to go to bed, it's time to rest and sleep, no matter whether it's 1 A.M. or 5 A.M. If you can't sleep, it's time for distraction and relaxation: reading, listening to music, or even watching TV. If you are having trouble sleeping, it is best not to focus your attention on the time. This is one of the bad sleeping habits that can aggravate insomnia. Looking at a clock every five or ten minutes while you are lying in bed or glancing at the clock to see what time it is each time you awaken during the night should be avoided.

TEMPERATURE

Make sure the room isn't too hot or too cold. Despite old beliefs, there is no evidence that an excessively cold room makes you sleep any better. In fact, cold feet can keep you awake; wear socks if that's a problem. An ideal temperature

for humans has not yet been determined; however, tempera-
tures below 55 or above 75 degrees Fahrenheit seem to
disturb sleep. Make sure the temperature in your bedroom is
comfortable for *you*. If it is not, consider installing an auxil-
iary heater, ceiling fan, air conditioner, or fan. If your temperature requirements differ from those of your sleeping partner,
find ways to arrive at a mutually satisfying arrangement.

Your room could be harmful to your sleep in other ways. If
you have an allergy, an open window could be bringing pollen
into your room, causing breathing problems. An old pillow
might be musty, causing you to sneeze, cough, or have itchy
eyes. You might need to clean under the bed and wash drapes,
blankets, and the bedspread to get rid of accumulated irritants.

While an open window or a draft can cause problems
for some people, others can't stand a closed-in room or air-
conditioning. Try your window open, try it closed, and see
which way is best for you.

Check the Simple Things

- Are your sheets fresh and comfortable?
- Is your blanket too light, too heavy, too scratchy, or
  too hot?
- Is your bedroom too hot or too cold and are your
  nightclothes uncomfortable?
- Do you have a dog or cat or bird scratching around in
  your bedroom at night?
- Are your mattress and pillow comfortable?

Change Psychological Conditioning

To reverse the insomnia-producing effects of negative conditioning and poor sleep habits, consider trying one or more of

the following strategies. These are often the most helpful and powerful strategies for coping with insomnia. They often require substantial patience and commitment, however, since most established habits are difficult—but not impossible—to overcome.

1 | *Create positive presleep rituals.* Try reading, taking a warm bath, listening to soft music, or anything else that relaxes and pleases you on a regular basis before going to bed. Avoid any activities that might be arousing, stimulating, or worry-producing unless they help you relax and get to sleep (e.g., sex).

2 | *Go to bed only when sleepy.* Don't use your bed for any other purposes other than sleep (and sex). Do not use your bed to work, read, watch television, or for any other purpose. Do these things in another room, at your desk, in a chair, or on the floor. When you finally feel sleepy, stop these activities and get into bed. This strategy will positively associate your bed with feeling sleepy over time.

3 | *Avoid trying to sleep.* By now, you should understand that the more you try to will yourself to sleep, the worse your problem will become. Remember, sleep is not a "task" to be performed. It requires a relaxed, calm, peaceful state, which usually means you are not willfully trying to do anything. Don't let yourself think about work, problems, goals, projects, or other important considerations. Save these for the daytime hours, when you are more alert and can possibly do something about them.

4 | *Establish a regular wake-up time* (regardless of how much sleep you get). One of the best ways to break an insomnia problem is to establish a consistent wake-up time and force yourself to stick to it seven days a week. For instance, set your alarm for 8 A.M. every day, and force yourself to get out of bed and get moving no matter how you feel at that time. Don't allow yourself to sleep later on weekends or on days when you don't have any responsibilities in the morning. By establishing a consistent wake-up time, you encourage your body and brain to adopt a consistent sleep-wake cycle. After awhile, this conditioned sleep-wake pattern will take over naturally on its own.

5 | *Set aside time to worry before going to bed.* If you tend to worry excessively whenever you try to sleep, set aside a period of time (no more than thirty minutes) to get all your worrying and thinking done before bedtime. Make a list of all your immediate problems and concerns. Write down one or two actions you could take tomorrow or in the near future to help resolve them. Then go to sleep knowing that you've given serious thought to each of these problems.

If you are lying in bed and begin to think of a new problem or difficulty that you forgot to consider, get out of bed, write it down, think about it for a minute, then get back into bed and forget about it. By all means, don't allow yourself to lie in bed thinking about it. If you do continue to think about it, force yourself to get out of bed until you are finished doing so. Some people find that keeping a small pad and pencil by their bedside is also helpful. If they awaken during the night with a critical new thought or idea, they can quickly jot it down, thereby avoiding any worry or anxiety that they will forget it come morning.

6 | *Limit time awake in bed.* Another very important strategy is to limit the time you spend awake in bed, particularly if you are unsuccessful at either getting to sleep or staying asleep. If you are unable to fall asleep, don't stay in your bed for more than ten to fifteen minutes. Get up, get out of bed, and do something productive or enjoyable (but not stressful or overly stimulating, such as working on your taxes or paying bills). Read, watch television, go to another room, and when you eventually feel drowsy, get back in bed and allow yourself to peacefully go to sleep. If ten to fifteen minutes go by again and you are still awake, get out of bed and repeat the strategy again.

7 | *Try sleeping in different locations.* Another useful strategy is to change your sleep environment. Since your main environment (usually your bedroom) can become negatively associated with sleeplessness, you may find that you sleep much better in nonfamiliar surroundings. Try sleeping in a guest room, on a couch in your living room, on the kitchen floor, or even a motel. This may sound strange, but it works for many people. If you find that this helps, it should be a clue that negative conditioning and negative associations are probably playing a role in your insomnia. Once you know this, you can apply some of the other strategies discussed in this section to reverse the negative patterns of thinking and behaving.

Avoid Alcohol, Caffeine, and Nicotine (Especially Late in the Day)

If you are having trouble sleeping, it is best to avoid alcohol, caffeine, and nicotine altogether. For example, the caffeine you ingest from one or two cups of coffee or tea can affect your brain for twelve to twenty-four hours. Similar effects can be produced by colas, chocolate, diet pills, and other caffeine-containing substances. If you can't stay away from these completely, try not to use them after lunch.

While alcohol may relax you and help you get to sleep, it can disturb nighttime sleep activity in your brain. This can cause you to wake up more frequently during the night and fail to obtain the deep sleep that is needed to refresh you. Smoking and other sources of nicotine (such as nicotine gum or patches) can also interfere with sleep. Nicotine is a powerful brain stimulant. When heavy smokers quit the habit, their sleep often improves in the long run.

Be careful not to abruptly withdraw any of these agents, especially if you have used them daily for months or years. Acute withdrawal reactions, and the arousal state that accompanies them, can often interfere with sleep and make your insomnia worse. For best results, consult your physician about how to gradually taper down and eventually discontinue these substances.

Don't Nap During the Day

While napping during the day may seem tempting—and even helpful—it can also work against you. Sleeping during the day makes it harder for you to get to sleep at night. This keeps you from establishing and maintaining a regular sleep-wake cycle, which is one of your best defenses against insomnia.

Exercise

Regular exercise (at least twenty minutes a day five to six days a week) can also improve your sleep. The amount and timing of exercise are both important for achieving this goal. In general, research has shown that the best time to exercise (for the purpose of improving sleep) is six hours prior to bedtime. Thus, for most people on a normal schedule, exercising late in the afternoon or early in the evening is best.

If you exercise early in the morning or too close to bedtime, this benefit may be lost. Exercise improves sleep by producing changes in chemical reactions throughout the body and the brain. Its effects may also be mediated by body temperature increases that occur with exercise. If you exercise too early in the day, these changes might wear off by bedtime. On the other hand, if you exercise too close to bedtime, these very same changes will be at their peak, and the resulting stimulation and body arousal may actually keep you awake.

If you are unable to exercise or are restricted from doing so for any reason, try taking a hot bath about two hours prior to bedtime. The resultant increase in body temperature may give you some of the same sleep benefits that others obtain from exercise.

Bedtime Snacks

Some people find that a bedtime snack helps them sleep. Others find eating or drinking too close to bedtime keeps them awake. Since both hunger and eating too much can interfere with sleep, you will have to experiment to see what works for you.

Which types of foods are most helpful? Research dating back to 1937 shows that warm milk, with or without cookies or other food, is beneficial. Warm milk may be better than cold because of the body temperature effect noted above. Turkey, high in tryptophan, is also helpful.

It is also best to avoid excessive liquids within one to two hours of sleeping. This is especially true if you have bladder problems, prostate problems, or other urinary tract conditions.

Shift Work

If you do shift work, you must pay more attention to your sleep routine than other people. Especially important is the need to protect your sleep environment and designated sleep time. Since most other people will be up and around during the time you need to sleep, you must keep them from interrupting you. Napping may be useful to catch up on lost sleep, but it is best to establish a daily sleep routine and do what is necessary to maintain it religiously.

You should also avoid using caffeine or other stimulants while on night duty, since these can interfere with your sleep the next day. Occasional use of sleeping pills might be needed, but you should avoid becoming dependent on frequent or daily use of these agents.

Learn to Deal with Stress

One of the best things you can do to prevent or eliminate insomnia is to learn how to deal with stress more effectively. Most people experience periods of anxiety, tension, worry, or irritability from time to time. These negative emotions can build up during the day and affect your ability to rest at night. In addition, unresolved conflicts and unexpressed emotions, which many people try to suppress or ignore, can come out at night in the form of troublesome dreams or the inability to relax when going to sleep.

Medications such as tranquilizers, antianxiety agents, and antidepressants, which many people use when under stress, can also disturb sleep. So can the increased use of cigarettes, caffeine, and alcohol, which often accompanies periods of emotional and psychological upheaval.

One way to mitigate stress is to use relaxation techniques. These include meditation, biofeedback, yoga, self-hypnosis, and other relaxation skills that can be used during the day or at bedtime. These techniques don't work for everyone, but you might want to give them a try. It's best to practice any of these techniques during daytime hours for several weeks before trying to use them at night. This will help you avoid premature failures or the disappointment that follows from excessively optimistic expectations.

Many people discover, however, that the best way to deal with stress is not by learning how to manage its symptoms, but by learning how to identify and deal with its underlying causes. Most stress management techniques, such as exercise, dietary changes, and relaxation procedures, are symptom-oriented approaches. If you're worried about finances or if you're having relationship conflicts both at home and at work, these coping strategies will usually be insufficient.

GIVE YOURSELF TIME TO WIND DOWN

The brain is not a switch. You cannot expect to work at full speed until 11 P.M. and fall asleep at 11:15. Take time to play, read a novel, or talk to your spouse or kids. Try not to wrestle with a problem or get into an argument just before going to bed.

An excellent way to wind down and get into the proper

frame of mind for sleep is a massage, especially if given by the loving hands of someone who cares about you.

REDUCING TENSION AND COPING WITH STRESS

A very important technique for aiding sleep is called progressive relaxation. Lying comfortably, you systematically focus on and consciously relax each part of your body starting with your toes, moving up through the ankles, calves, knees, all the way up to the head. Don't forget to visualize the inner organs relaxing when you're at the belly. And don't forget the eyes, ears, and brain. Feel the tissues softening, becoming warm, heavy, and compliant to the idea of deep relaxation. For a more detailed exploration of the preceding suggestions, refer to page 49.

PART III

Stress

9

What Is Stress?

Stress is best described as a group of body-wide, nonspecific responses induced by any number of situations or events. Just staying alive creates demands on the body for life-maintaining energy; even while we are asleep, our bodies continue to function. So by this definition, stress is a fundamental part of being alive and should not be avoided. The trick is to ensure that the degree of stress we experience is such that life is a joy, not a drag.

From this perspective, energy usage is one characteristic of stress. Another characteristic is lack of specificity. Any demands made upon us in daily life bring about certain reactions in the body. These same reactions occur under a whole range of different conditions, both physical and emotional—from hot and cold to joy and sorrow. As aware, feeling people, we probably make a big distinction between the pain caused by the loss of a loved one and the pain caused by the temperature dropping too fast; but the nature of the demand is unimportant at the biological level. To the body, it's all the same because the stress response is always the same. Nerve signals are sent from the brain to several glands, and these react by secreting hormones to cope with the task ahead. So stress is not just worry and strain. It is a keynote of life, with all its ups and downs. A new and exciting love can cause us as much stress as a cranky boss.

The wide array of triggers that elicit the stress response are known as stressors. There are many potential stressors, such as changes (vacation, marriage, divorce, a new job, and so on); any intense emotion, such as fear or anger; or fatigue, physical injury, surgery, temperature extremes, noise, crowding, or illness.

Change is one of the most powerful stressors. Any kind of change in our lives, even one perceived as positive, requires an adaptation to a new set of circumstances. Getting married, getting divorced, entering college, and graduating from college all require adaptation and thus are all stressors. The effects of stressors are cumulative. The more stressors in one's life at any given time, the higher the stress levels will be.

No two people are exactly alike as to which aspects of daily life will increase their stress levels. The identical life situation might be quite pleasant to one person while extremely stressful to another. In a general sense, a situation will be a stressor if it is perceived as threatening to our well-being or requiring adjustment in any way. It is the perception of each situation that makes it either stressful or not, so almost any event or situation can be a stressor.

How Stress Contributes to Illness

There is a definite relationship between stress and illness. Although the exact nature of that relationship is not yet understood, a number of ideas have been suggested. Early theories tried to connect different illnesses with specific types of emotional conflict or personality and body types.

Hans Selye maintains that the biological reactions accompanying adaptation to stress result in both short- and long-term adverse physical changes. He calls these changes "diseases of adaptation," since they are the outcome of a system of defenses against threatening stimuli. The disease process is thought to arise as a result of factors such as the physiological effect of certain hormones from the adrenal and pituitary glands, the impact of the inflammation process, and a general state of lowered resistance. The actual disease that manifests itself depends on a range of factors, including genetics, physical weakness, and even specifically learned bodily responses.

This helps explain the effects of life changes or events on health. Life changes require adjustments that might produce physiological reactions. Moreover, sustained and unsuccessful attempts at coping with change can eventually lower bodily resistance, thus enhancing the probability of illness. The more frequent and severe the life changes we experience, the more likely we are to become ill. As examples, consider the following:

- **Heart disease.** Stress contributes to heart disease in many ways. During periods of stress, the blood pressure rises and the pulse increases, placing an increased burden on the heart. Stress includes changes in blood chemistry, such as elevated cholesterol levels, that promote atherosclerosis. Finally, the coronary arteries that supply blood to the heart muscle itself narrow, reducing the amount of oxygen available to the heart muscle.

- **Infectious diseases.** Excessive stress reduces the effectiveness of the immune response and thus increases the risk of infection. Many people find that they experience colds mostly during stressful periods. Similarly, both oral and genital herpes attacks tend to develop during periods of high stress.

- **Cancer.** As with infectious diseases, excessive stress increases the risk of cancer by reducing the efficiency of the immune system. In every person, cells become cancerous from time to time. If the immune system is working properly, these cancerous cells are usually destroyed quickly.

- **Digestive disorders.** The sympathetic nervous system, which is activated during periods of stress, reduces production of most digestive juices, except for stomach acid. Food lies in the stomach, the acid builds up in response to the presence of the food, causing indigestion. In time, this acid can erode the wall of the stomach or intestine, causing an ulcer. Indigestion is a very common sign of excessive stress. Further, many people overeat or undereat during stressful periods, contributing to weight-management problems.

- **Skin disorders.** The impact of excessive stress on skin has long been recognized. Two very obvious effects are the appearance of rashes and premature aging. Stress produces rashes by modifying the activity of the immune mechanism. Premature aging of the skin results from stress-induced narrowing of the small blood vessels supplying food and oxygen to the skin cells.

Herbs, Lifestyle, and Stress Management

A well-balanced stress management program must address all aspects of life, and while herbal remedies will only fulfill some aspects, they are vital. It can help to group the many factors to be considered into four categories.

1 | *Physiological and metabolic factors.* This involves addressing factors affecting the inner workings of the body through nutrition, herbs, and drugs, when necessary. Herbal medicines offer an effective but gentle way to address some of the physiological and biochemical issues involved in stress management ranging from direct support of the adrenal glands to easing the plethora of symptoms that can result from the stress response.

2 | *Structural factors.* Here techniques are considered that address structural integration. This includes the manipulative therapies such as osteopathy, chiropractic, and all varieties of massage. Personal lifestyle will contribute exercise, dance, or any expression of bodily vitality. Relaxation techniques are invaluable.

3 | *Emotional and mental factors.* Psychological techniques are important for identifying and treating emotional and mental factors in health and disease. All the branches of psychotherapy are involved here, but especially the more holistically oriented approaches of humanistic and transpersonal psychology. A conscious and free-flowing emotional life is fundamental to achieving any inner harmony. This does not mean that everyone must get involved in depth psychology but that attention be given in the appropriate form for an individual's emotional needs.

4 | *Spirituality.* Spiritual factors in human healing are becoming increasingly recognized by materialistic

Western medicine. There are meditative and prayer-based techniques where the person aligns his or her being with a higher spirit, or those where a practitioner works with the energy body of a patient. Some openness to spirituality is vital and it might take the form of an uplifting sunset, being touched by poetry or art, belief in a religion, or simply joy in being alive.

Gardening, Tree Hugging, and Stress Management

If we get a bit creative it is easy to see how herbalism fits into a broad holistic context. The role of herbs need not be limited to their ingestion. This is a perfect excuse to get into the garden, walk in the woods, and literally "smell the roses!"

Chamomile is a very useful relaxing herb, combining a pleasant flavor with a range of relevant properties. Before the Victorians developed the grass lawn (a major cause of stress for some people!), lawns were made up of varieties of herbs that could cope with being trampled upon, and chamomile was one of these. A chamomile lawn makes a wonderfully restful place where you can lie on the herbs, relaxing the body while the wonderful aroma wafts around you. If the lawn is one you grew yourself, there are the added stress-reducers of exercise and a sense of fulfillment.

A specific variety of chamomile must be used: *Chamoemelum nobile*, "Treneague," is an apple-scented, nonflowering variety that works well, but the ordinary Roman chamomile saved from seed, which is less expensive, can also be used. Prepare the soil and then broadcast the seed. Cover with a thin layer of soil and keep moist but not wet. Once seedlings appear and have at least two sets of leaves, thin them out to about three inches apart. Don't walk on them until they are beginning to bind together. Remove most flower heads, as they appear to ensure leaf vigor, but allow occasional flowers to remain, as they form part of the lawn's charm. Avoid having a chamomile lawn bordering on a grass or wild garden, as creeping weeds will soon invade the lawn and uprooting them will disturb the shallow-rooted chamomile plants. A surround of stone, brick, or paving slabs is ideal.

If a very broad view is taken of herbalism, seeing it as an exploration of humanity's relationship with the plant world, some unusual healing possibilities present themselves. In recent years, researchers from several disciplines have begun investigating the benefits of contacts with plants, especially trees. In studies of the stress-reducing effects of nature, people recovered more quickly and completely from stress when exposed to plant-rich natural settings. This was indicated by lower blood pressure, heart rate, muscle tension, and skin conductance. Psychological recovery was also facilitated with measurable reductions of fear and anger and increases in positive feelings. Physiological findings indicated that the nature settings produced significant recovery from stress in only four to six minutes. This rapid recovery highlights the importance of plants for city dwellers who are often stressed out by commuting and work pressures.

In a comparison of the hospital records of gall bladder surgery patients who had window views of either a small stand of trees or a brick building wall, it was found that those with the view of trees had shorter postoperative hospital stays, required fewer potent drugs for pain, and received fewer negative staff evaluations about their conditions than those with the wall view.

10

Green Medicine to Relieve Stress

Herbs can help the body and mind cope with the stress response in a number of ways, in addition to the rather simplistic ones of stimulation and relaxation. In Western herbalism today, it is common to differentiate between groups of herbs that have similar physiological effects on people. Herbs that act on the nervous system are collectively called *nervines*, and are grouped into nervine tonics, nervine relaxants, and nervine stimulants. There are also muscle-relaxing antispasmodics and sleep-inducers known as *hypnotics*. Of most direct relevance for stress management are the *adaptogenic* herbs.

Types of Herbs

Adaptogens

As we approach the twenty-first century, we live in a world of stress, pollution, lack of meaning, and lack of purpose. In the face of such a cultural alienation from nature, the plethora of diseases assailing the "civilized" world should come as no surprise. To heal these ills, the underlying causes must first be addressed and these causes are not only within the individual but within our culture as a whole. When a health problem is related to lowered resistance due to the impact of a hostile environment, we must first heal the hostile environment. In other words, even if there were a remedy that offered individuals protection against toxic chemicals, it would be preferable to remove the toxic chemical from the environment. This makes economic sense, is the right stance in Hippocratic terms, and is right action in spiritual terms.

When attention is given to appropriate support for the body under stressful conditions, nature comes to our rescue. Technically, what is needed is an increase in nonspecific resistance to damaging man-made factors and illnesses. A range of herbal remedies are coming to light that do this. Soviet scientists coined the term "adaptogens" to describe herbs that produce this wonderful increase in resistance and vitality, defining them like this:

- An adaptogen must show a nonspecific activity, i.e., increase in power of resistance against physical, chemical, or biological noxious agents.

- An adaptogen must have a normalizing influence independent of the nature of the pathological state.

- An adaptogen must be innocuous and must not influence normal body functions more than required.

In this sense, adaptogens reinforce the nonspecific power of resistance against stressors, increase general capacities to withstand situations of stress, and hence guard against disease caused by overstress of the organism. The general aim of adaptogen treatment is a reduction of stress reactions during the alarm phase of the stress response, prevention or at least delaying of the state of exhaustion, and hence a certain level of protection against long-term stress.

A number of herbs that can be described as adaptogens include ginseng, Siberian ginseng, ashwaganda, shiitake, and schizandra. It is worth looking at the evidence for adaptogenicity in a little depth. Rather than exploring the background for all these adaptogenic herbs, we will focus on Siberian ginseng.

SIBERIAN GINSENG (*Eleutherococcus senticosus*)

Siberian ginseng, one of the most remarkable of adaptogenic plants, has a wide range of uses and very low toxicity. There has been a great deal of excellent clinical and laboratory research conducted in the Soviet Union, where Professor Brehkman and his team have been studying the herb for over thirty years. Large-scale clinical trials have been undertaken on both healthy and sick people with more than 1,000 published research papers devoted to its application, the mechanism of action, and investigation of its active principles.

Pharmacological research suggests that the active principle of the adaptogenic plants—the *eleutherosides* from Siberian ginseng and the *panaxosides* from ginseng—are *saponin glycosides,* which increase the general nonspecific resistance of the body to a whole range of diverse chemical, physical, psychological, and biological factors. Its safety and ability to increase the resistance of the normal human body to extreme conditions make Siberian ginseng a remedy of great importance.

Studies on Siberian ginseng provide some of the best clinical trials done on herbal medicines so far. Large numbers of people including control groups were involved in these studies. Between 1973 and 1975, 1,200 drivers from the Volga automobile plant were given 8 to 12 mg of Siberian ginseng extract daily with tea for two months each year in the spring and autumn. By the end of the experiment, illness among the drivers had *decreased* by 20 to 30 percent, while the total disease incidence among other workers at the plant *increased* by 20 percent. Based on these results, the authorities at the factory undertook a mass program of preventive medicine with the herb in the winter of 1975. It was included in the diet as Siberian ginseng sugar at a per day dose of 2 ml. Altogether, 13,096 persons were engaged in the experiment. The overall disease incidence dropped by 30 to 35 percent as compared to a control group that did not use the remedy.

In another clinical trial, a group of fifty-four miners received the extract before the beginning of their shift daily in June and July of 1976. The number of people reporting sick dropped by 33.3 percent and the number of days lost through illness dropped by 45.6 percent. Reduction of the incidence of influenza and acute respiratory diseases was particularly impressive. In a strict medical sense, Siberian ginseng is an adrenal stimulant and not an antiviral remedy. However, the Russians have accumulated much data on the anti-influenzal effect of the herb as well. Such findings imply that either it possesses an invigorating and tonic action on natural immunity or it has direct antivirus activity.

Conditions shown to improve with Siberian ginseng

There is an ever-lengthening list of pathologies that have been demonstrated to improve with the use of this adaptogen. Here is a short list based on published results:

- Neurasthenia
- Hypertension
- Chronic gastritis

- Diabetes
- Atherosclerosis
- Tuberculosis
- Brain injuries
- Infectious diseases

Cancer

Siberian ginseng is also being used in Russia for the postoperative treatment of cancer patients. Not only does it speed postoperative recovery, but it ameliorates the stress response that can aggravate metastasis, the spreading of cancer cells around the body. The ability of Siberian ginseng to potentiate antitumor immunity has also been discovered recently. It increases antineoplastic white blood cells (natural "killer cells") and induces the synthesis of γ-interferon by leukocytes. It is well known that stress decreases the activity of the immune system and particularly that of the natural killer cells. An obvious association exists here on a biochemical level between stress, immune function, and the herb Siberian ginseng.

In these times of pollution and exposure to strange and dangerous chemicals, this fascinating plan may prove of vital help as it also reduces the toxic impact of a number of chemical compounds. In laboratory tests, Siberian ginseng was shown to decrease the sensitivity of mice and rats to the toxicity of a range of chemicals. When the animals were treated with cytotoxic drugs combined with Siberian ginseng, they lost less weight and their white blood count was higher than in the animals treated with the drugs alone. The implications for using this herb as support in anticancer chemotherapy are clear and exciting.

A fundamental problem with the use of cytotoxic drugs in cancer therapy is that they destroy not only cancer cells but healthy ones as well. In the test, lethal doses of the drugs resulted in the animals' death, but when Siberian ginseng and drugs were used in combination, the death rate dropped. In a group of mice given thiophosphamide in a dose of 16 mg/kg, 53 percent of the animals died. After administering combined Siberian ginseng and thiophosphamide, only 15 percent of the animals died. Similar results were obtained in a group of animals given ethymidin in a dose of 1.5 mg/kg. Thirty percent so treated died, while all those receiving both the herb and drug remained alive.

Siberian ginseng also appears able to reduce the narcotic effects of a number of drugs. For example, it shortens the duration of sleep induced by sedatives. It may also prove useful for prophylactic and therapeutic applications in acute and chronic poisoning with some insecticides and industrial poisons. This ability of Siberian ginseng is linked with its ability to activate the body's own metabolic system for inactivating toxins. Therefore, Russian pharmacologists advise the use of the extract in different drug formulae to reduce their inherent toxicity.

It is clear that Siberian ginseng is a very special remedy indeed. It can increase individual resistance to the whole spectrum of factors that contribute to stress reactions and exhaustion. Apparently, the herb will help whether the stress is from extremes of weather or from psychological exhaustion. Its universal properties make this herb one of the most efficacious and promising medicines for increasing hardiness against the many stresses of contemporary life.

Nervines

A nervine is a plant that has an effect upon the nervous system in some way: there are nervine tonics, nervine relaxants, and nervine stimulants. Remember that any successful treatment of nervous system problems with herbs must involve treating the whole body, heart, and mind, not simply the signs of agitation and worry. Of course, the agitation can be reduced greatly by the appropriate herbs, but the whole system must be strengthened in the face of the storm as well.

NERVINE TONICS

Perhaps the most helpful contribution herbal medicine can make is to strengthen and "feed" the nervous system. In cases of shock, stress, or nervous debility, the nervine tonics strengthen and restore the tissues directly. On the other hand, they can contribute to the healing of damaged nervous tissue, whether this is due to a pathological process or physical trauma. This invaluable group of remedies is best exemplified by oats. Ginkgo is an important tonic for the nervous system but appears to work via its vasodilating action on the blood

---

MILD RELAXING NERVINES

Balm	Chamomile	Lavender
Black cohosh	Hyssop	Red clover

MEDIUM RELAXING NERVINES

Damiana	Motherwort	Skullcap
Linden	Mugwort	St. John's wort
Lobelia	Pulsatilla	Vervain

STRONG RELAXING NERVINES

California poppy	Passionflower	Wild lettuce
Hops	Valerian	

vessels of the brain, thereby increasing oxygen availability to brain cells. Other nervine tonics can have, in addition, a relaxing effect. Skullcap is often the most effective, particularly for problems related to stress.

NERVINE RELAXANTS

This group of nervines are extremely useful in our times of stress and confusion, alleviating many of the accompanying symptoms. They should always be used in a broad holistic way, not simply to tranquilize. Too much tranquilizing, even that achieved through herbal medication, can in time deplete and weigh heavily on the whole nervous system.

Many of the nervine relaxants also have other properties and can be selected to aid in related problems. This is one of the great benefits of using herbal remedies to help in stress and anxiety problems. The physical symptoms that often accompany anxiety may be treated with herbs that work on the anxiety itself. They can also be grouped in terms of their relative strength, bearing in mind that not all people respond to herbs in the same way.

Since each system of the body has plants that are particularly suited to it, relaxing nervines can be selected based on their affinity for the various systems.

- **Circulatory system.** Balm, linden, and motherwort are generally helpful to the cardiovascular system. However, most remedies that reduce overactivity in the nervous system will aid the heart and ameliorate problems such as high blood pressure.

- **Respiratory system.** Most sedatives will help in asthma, but black cohosh, lobelia, motherwort, and wild lettuce are especially helpful.

- **Digestive system.** All the relaxing and antispasmodic remedies may be of value here to ease colic, but sedatives that actively aid digestion include balm, chamomile, and lavender.

- **Reproductive system.** Black cohosh, blue cohosh, crampbark, motherwort, and wild lettuce all have an affinity for this system.

- **Muscles and skeleton.** All sedative remedies will ease muscular tension and thus pain in this complex system. Black cohosh is especially helpful.

- **Nervous system.** All the remedies mentioned above relate here.

- **Skin.** All these nervines may help the skin in an indirect way, but the following herbs are especially beneficial for the skin: red clover, St. John's wort, pulsatilla, and black cohosh.

While any of the above nervines will be generally relaxing, another way to select the herb (or herbs) that will prove most appropriate is to take into account their other properties. The range of options and the various subtleties can be daunting and complex, but as examples consider the list below. It combines the need for relaxation with other common symptoms as an indication for relevant herbs.

- **Delayed menstruation.** Black cohosh, motherwort, mugwort.

- **Diarrhea.** Black haw, crampbark, hops, linden.

- **Muscle tightness.** Black cohosh, black haw, crampbark, hops, lavender, lobelia, valerian.

- **Colic.** Balm, black haw, chamomile, hops, hyssop, lavender, linden, mugwort, valerian.

- **Sinus congestion.** Chamomile, hyssop, linden.
- **Heartburn.** Balm, chamomile, linden.
- **Arthritis.** Black cohosh, Jamaican dogwood.
- **Skin problems.** Red clover.
- **Flatulence.** Balm, chamomile, hops, hyssop, lavender, motherwort, mugwort, valerian.
- **Hypertension.** Linden, motherwort, passionflower, skullcap, valerian.
- **Asthma.** Lobelia, motherwort, wild cherry bark, wild lettuce.
- **Menstrual cramps.** Black cohosh, blue cohosh, crampbark, motherwort, skullcap, valerian, wild lettuce.

NERVINE STIMULANTS

Direct stimulation of the nervous tissue is not often needed in our times of hyperactivity. It is usually more appropriate to stimulate the body's innate vitality with the help of nervine or bitter tonics, which work by augmenting bodily harmony and thus have a much deeper and longer-lasting effect than nervine stimulants. In the last century, much more emphasis was placed by herbalists upon stimulant herbs. It is, perhaps, a sign of the times that our world is supplying us with more than enough stimulus.

When direct nervine stimulation is indicated, an herb to use is kola nut, although guarana, coffee, maté, and tea should also be remembered. A problem with these commonly used stimulants is that they have a number of side effects and can themselves be involved in aggravating psychological problems such as anxiety and tension.

Some of the herbs rich in volatile oils are also valuable

stimulants; among them the commonest and best are rosemary and peppermint.

Antispasmodics

In addition to the herbs that work directly on the nervous system, the antispasmodic herbs—which affect the peripheral nerves and the muscle tissue—can have an indirect relaxing effect on the body. When the physical body is at ease, a relaxed psyche follows. Many of the nervine relaxants have this antispasmodic action. The antispasmodics relax the autonomic nervous system and not necessarily the central nervous system. This allows a physical relaxation of muscles without a sedative effect upon consciousness.

ANTISPASMODICS

Balm	Jamaican dogwood	Roman chamomile
Black cohosh		
Black haw	Lavender	Rosemary
Bugleweed	Licorice	Skullcap
California poppy	Linden	Skunk cabbage
	Lobelia	St. John's wort
Catmint	Motherwort	Sundew
Celery seed	Mugwort	Thyme
Chamomile	Mullein	Valerian
Crampbark	Parsley	Wild cherry
Damiana	Pasque flower	Wild lettuce
Ginger	Passionflower	Wild yam
Hyssop	Peppermint	
Hops	Red clover	

Listed below are some common conditions and the appropriate antispasmodic herbs for relieving them:

- **Delayed menstruation.** Black cohosh, caraway, motherwort, mugwort, pennyroyal.

- **Diarrhea.** Black haw, bugleweed, crampbark, ground ivy, hops, linden, red sage, rosemary, St. John's wort, wild cherry.

- **Muscle tightness.** Black cohosh, black haw, crampbark, hops, lavender, lobelia, valerian.

- **Colic.** Angelica, aniseed, balm, caraway, cardamom, catnip, chamomile, dill, fennel, fenugreek, ginger, hops, hyssop, lavender, motherwort, mugwort, parsley, pennyroyal, peppermint, red sage, Roman chamomile, rosemary, thyme, valerian, vervain, wild carrot.

- **Sinus congestion.** Betony, catmint, chamomile, coltsfoot, elder, fenugreek, ginger, hyssop, lavender, linden, mullein, peppermint, red sage, thyme.

- **Heartburn.** Coltsfoot, fenugreek, licorice, mullein.

- **Arthritis.** Angelica, black cohosh, celery seed, elder, lavender, licorice, linden, wild yam.

- **Skin problems.** Black cohosh, red clover.

- **Flatulence.** Balm, chamomile, hops, hyssop, lavender, motherwort, mugwort, valerian.

- **Hypertension.** Linden, motherwort, passionflower, skullcap, valerian.

- **Asthma.** Lobelia, motherwort, wild cherry bark, wild lettuce.

- **Menstrual cramps.** Black cohosh, black haw, crampbark, motherwort, skullcap, valerian, wild lettuce.

Hypnotics

Hypnotics are herbal remedies that will help to induce a deep and healing state of sleep. They have nothing at all to do with hypnotic trances. Herbs that promote sleep have modes of action that vary from mild, muscle-relaxing properties, through volatile oils that ease psychological tensions, to remedies that contain strong alkaloids that work directly on the central nervous system and put you to sleep. Some of the most effective plant hypnotics are illegal for the very reason of their effectiveness. This includes the whole range of opium poppy derivatives. The remedies mentioned here are entirely safe and have no addictive properties. When treating sleep problems, hypnotic herbs should always be used in conjunction with attention to relaxation, diet, and lifestyle.

Each system of the body has plants that are particularly suited to it, some of which are hypnotics of varying strength. It is safe to say, however, that all the hypnotic remedies can help the whole body in that sleep is such a vital health process.

- **Circulatory system.** Motherwort, linden, balm. They are all in the milder group.

- **Respiratory system.** All the hypnotics can help as antispasmodics in conditions such as asthma, if used at the right dose. Wild lettuce eases irritable coughs.

MILD HYPNOTICS	MEDIUM HYPNOTICS	STRONG HYPNOTICS
Chamomile	California poppy	Hops
Linden	Motherwort	Jamaican dogwood
Mugwort	Pulsatilla	Passionflower
	Skullcap	Pulsatilla
		Valerian
		Wild lettuce

- **Digestive system.** The relaxing nervines and carminatives are important, especially balm, chamomile, hops, and valerian. The antispasmodic herbs will help with intestinal colic, for example, hops, Jamaican dogwood, passionflower, and valerian.

- **Muscles and skeleton.** All hypnotics will aid in reducing muscle tension and even the pain associated with problems in this system. They may be used internally or as lotions. Especially important are Jamaican dogwood and valerian.

- **Skin.** Chamomile and cowslip are healing, but otherwise the value of hypnotics here is to ensure that the body has a good recuperative rest each night.

Bach Flower Remedies

This unique healing system consists of essences made from thirty-eight different flowers, each having a specific action upon a certain mental attitude. Just as the body has its own self-healing properties regarding diseases and wounds, the mind and spirit have their own self-healing capacities, which the Bach Flower Remedies stimulate. The remedies used are all prepared from the flowers of wild plants, bushes, and trees, and none of them is harmful or habit-forming.

They are used for worry, apprehension, hopelessness, irritability, and so on, because these states of mind or moods hinder recovery of health, retard convalescence, and often are the underlying causes of sickness and disease. A long-continued worry or fear depletes one's vitality.

It is important to identify the nature of the individual's unique "patterns" before selecting the appropriate remedy. Consider the person's attitudes, feelings, worries, indecision, timidity, vexations, resentment, possessiveness, hopelessness, lethargy, hatred, overpowering or demanding nature, intolerance, tenseness, etc., and, most importantly, the reason behind the apprehension, worry, and fear. Only then can the correct remedy or remedies be determined.

AGRIMONY. Those who suffer inner torture, which they try to hide behind a facade of cheerfulness. Often used as a remedy for alcoholism.

ASPEN. Apprehension, the feeling that something dreadful is going to happen without knowing why. Anxiety for no known reason.

BEECH. Critical and intolerant of others. Arrogant.

CENTAURY. Weakness of will; those who let themselves be exploited or imposed upon; they have difficulty in saying "no." A human doormat.

CERATO. Those who doubt their own judgment and intuition, always seeking the advice of others. Often influenced and misguided.

CHERRY PLUM. Uncontrolled, irrational thoughts. Fear of losing control and doing something terrible, fear of "going crazy." Uncontrolled bursts of temper. Impulsively suicidal.

CHESTNUT BUD. Refusal to learn by experience; continually repeating the same mistakes.

CHICORY. Overly possessive, demands respect or attention, likes others to conform to their standards. Makes martyr of oneself. Interferes and manipulates.

CLEMATIS. Indifferent, inattentive, daydreaming, absent-minded. Mental escapist from reality.

CRAB APPLE. "The Cleanser Flower." Feels unclean or ashamed of ailments. Self-disgust/hatred. House proud.

ELM. Temporarily overcome by inadequacy or responsibility, though normally very capable.

GENTIAN. Despondent. Easily discouraged and rejected. Skeptical, pessimistic. Depression, when its cause is known.

GORSE. Desperate, without hope: "Oh, what's the use?" Defeatism.

HEATHER. People who are obsessed with their own troubles and experiences. Talkative bores, poor listeners.

HOLLY. For those who are jealous, envious, revengeful, and suspicious. Those who hate.

HONEYSUCKLE. For those with nostalgia who constantly dwell in the past. Homesickness.

HORNBEAM. "Monday morning" feeling, but once started, task is usually fulfilled. Mentally tired. Procrastination.

IMPATIENS. Impatience, irritability. Reacts in an exaggerated manner.

LARCH. Despondency due to lack of self-confidence; expectation of failure, so fails to make the attempt. Feels inferior, yet has the ability.

MIMULUS. Fear of known things, fear of the world. Shyness, timidity, bashfulness.

MUSTARD. Dark cloud of depression that descends for no known reason, which can lift just as suddenly, making one downcast, saddened, and low.

OAK. Brave determined type. Struggles on in illness and against adversity despite setbacks. Plodders, never resting.

OLIVE. Drained of energy, everything an effort. Physically fatigued.

PINE. Feelings of guilt. Blames oneself for the mistakes of others. Feels unworthy.

RED CHESTNUT. Excessive care of and concern for others, especially those held dear.

ROCK ROSE. Alarmed, panicky, full of trepidation.

ROCK WATER. For those who are hard on themselves and often overwork. Rigid, self-denying, ascetic.

SCLERANTHUS. Uncertainty, indecision, vacillation. Fluctuating moods.

STAR OF BETHLEHEM. For all the effects of upsetting news or fright following an accident. For release from trauma, no matter how old it is.

SWEET CHESTNUT. Absolute dejection. Feels as if one has reached the limits of what one can stand.

VERVAIN. Overenthusiasm, overeffort, straining. Fanatical and highly strung. Incensed and frustrated by injustices.

VINE. Dominating/inflexible/ambitious/tyrannical/autocratic. Arrogant pride. Considered to be good leaders.

WALNUT. Protection remedy against powerful influences; helps adjustment to any transition or change, e.g., puberty, menopause, divorce, new surroundings. Unlike Centaury, the person knows what he wants but is easily influenced by other people to do something else.

WATER VIOLET. Proud, reserved, sedate types, sometimes feel "superior." Little emotional involvement but reliable, dependent.

WHITE CHESTNUT. Persistent unwanted thoughts. Preoccupation with some worry or episode. Mental arguments. Constant inner dialogue.

WILD OAT. Helps determine one's intended path of life.

WILD ROSE. Resignation, apathy. Drifters who accept their lot, making little or no effort for improvement; lacks ambition.

WILLOW. Resentment and bitterness with "not fair" and "poor me" attitude.

RESCUE REMEDY. Dr. Bach combined five specific remedies (cherry plum, clematis, impatiens, rock rose, star of Bethlehem) to formulate an emergency composite that he called Rescue Remedy. Its purpose is to comfort, reassure, and calm those who have received upsetting news or have experienced a trauma. Rescue Remedy is invaluable to keep on hand for immediate emergency use; however, it does not take the place of medical attention. It is taken orally (4 drops) in a glass of water but can also be applied externally either in liquid or cream form.

The Bach Remedies are benign in their action without unpleasant side effects; thus, they can be taken by anyone. Stock concentrate remedies will keep indefinitely; a 10 ml concentrate bottle will make approximately sixty treatment bottles. More than one remedy can be taken at the same time. Place 2 drops of each chosen remedy in a glass of water and sip at intervals during the day or prepare a treatment bottle: fill a 1-fluid-ounce dropper bottle with spring water, add 2 drops of each chosen remedy, and place 4 drops of this mixture directly on the tongue at least four times a day.

11

Herbal Treatments for Stress

If a period of stress is predictably about to occur, it can be prepared for ahead of time, as herbs, diet, and any appropriate lifestyle changes will minimize the impact. Nervine relaxants can be used regularly as gentle soothing remedies. The following herbs can be taken as teas, cold drinks, infused in massage oil, or used in relaxing footbaths or full baths.

Balm	Linden	Red Clover
Chamomile	Mugwort	Skullcap
Lavender	Oats	St. John's wort

A daily supplement of vitamin B complex and vitamin C is also suggested. By using herbs and improving the diet, you are responding to stress in a healthy way, and the impact of the various stressors can be ameliorated. Relaxation exercises and an honest reevaluation of both lifestyle and life goals are invaluable. This is not always easy, but remember that people can change, change their lives, and reevaluate their choices.

The line between chronic stress and the daily levels we all seem to put up with is fuzzy. A gentle soul with a delicate constitution will cross the line sooner than a stronger person who copes well. Neither of these extremes is better than the other; they merely reflect the fact that we live in a world of human diversity. That's sometimes a joy and sometimes an actual cause of stress! The advice given above holds for chronic stress, but in addition, adaptogens become pivotal in this situation. Important examples are ginseng, Siberian ginseng, and ashwaganda.

Perhaps Siberian ginseng is the most highly recommended because it has no toxicity and lacks the stimulating effects some people experience with Korean or American ginseng. The usual dosage of the tincture is ½ to ¾ teaspoon three times a day. Commercial products are increasingly made from a highly concentrated dry extract. First they are extracted using a liquid, which is dried to a powder and then made into tablets. An equivalent dosage using a solid extract concentrated at a ratio of 20:1 would by 100 to 200 mg. The recommended regime is usually for a six-week course followed by a two-week break. This regime can be repeated for as long as is necessary.

In addition to adaptogens, every attention must be given to general health as the body will often show its stress through some physical symptom. This may be a long-standing complaint that gets worse, an old problem that reappears, or just a speeding of the aging process.

There are times in most people's lives when things get to be too much and the pain of existence builds to a crescendo. Immediate herbal relief may be needed in a whole range of traumatic situations—from being involved in a car accident to some personal emotional crisis. In all cases, herbs will take the edge off the trauma but will rarely remove it. At such times, herbs can be only an aid, just one element of the approach taken to deal with the difficulties being faced. This approach may also include seeking help from a health professional, going on vacation or a retreat, or even checking into a hospital.

The plants that are capable of easing intense stress are considered dangerous in our society, and because they are restricted drugs, they will not be discussed here. However, in addition to the herbs previously mentioned, the following remedies might be considered: passionflower, valerian, wild lettuce.

Notice the dosage here (1 teaspoon of tincture as needed). This is a recognition that the stress response has a cyclical nature and each person will find certain times of the day more challenging than others. As this is largely symptomatic medication, it may be increased until the desired relief is experienced. The dosage regime may be altered as necessary, varying time of day and quantity of dose to suit individual needs. For example, this may be a large dose first thing in the morning, or smaller amounts at frequent intervals throughout the day. The patient's experience is the guiding principle here. Always treat the human being and not the theory about the disease.

Basic Stress Formula

- 2 parts skullcap
- 2 parts valerian
- 1 part oats

Take 1 teaspoon of tincture as needed.

A possible prescription for acute stress associated with indigestion and palpitations:

- 2 parts skullcap
- 2 parts valerian
- 1 part motherwort
- 1 part chamomile
- 1 part mugwort

Take 1 teaspoon of tincture as needed. The motherwort supports relaxation but also has a specific calming impact on palpitations.

Anxiety

When the level of stress goes beyond the point of being a healthy stimulant and starts to adversely affect our health, it often takes the form of anxiety. It might surface as fear, apprehension, or a wide range of bodily symptoms. These are most prominent in the early stages of the illness and represent a reasonable reaction to the onset of illness and the related uncertainties.

Generalized anxiety disorder (GAD) is much more than the normal anxiety people experience day to day. It is chronic and exaggerated worry and tension, even though nothing seems to provoke it. Having this disorder means always anticipating disaster, often worrying excessively about health, money, family, or work. Sometimes, though, the source of the worry is hard to pinpoint. Simply the thought of getting through the day might provoke anxiety. People with GAD can't seem to shake their concerns, even though they usually realize that their anxiety is more intense than the situation warrants. They also seem unable to relax and have trouble falling or staying asleep. Their worries are accompanied by any of the physical symptoms listed on the following pages.

There may be no recognizable basis for the fear or feeling of threat, or the actual stimulus may be completely out of proportion to the emotion it provokes. Nevertheless, the symptoms it provokes are very real. For some people, anxiety takes the form of recurrent attacks that, though they occur unpredictably, may become associated with specific situations. They start with a sudden, intense apprehension, often combined with a feeling of impending doom and sometimes with feelings of unreality. Any of the symptoms described below may occur. An "anticipatory fear" or loss of control often develops, so that the person experiencing the attack becomes afraid of, for example, being left alone in a public place. The anticipatory fear may itself precipitate other symptoms that escalate the attack.

People with panic disorder have feelings of terror that strike suddenly and repeatedly with no warning. They can't predict when an attack will occur, and many develop intense anxiety between episodes, worrying when and where the next one will strike. In between times there is a persistent, lingering worry that another attack could come any minute. While most attacks average a couple of minutes, occasionally they can go on for up to ten minutes. In rare cases, they may last an hour or more.

Symptoms of Anxiety

There are a whole range of reactions associated with anxiety.*

Anxious mood. Worrying, apprehension, anticipation of the worst, irritability.

The remedies. The herbal approaches described in the following section will be generally helpful, but the Bach Flower Remedies are especially relevant. For example, aspen and rock rose are indicated in states of apprehension.

Fear. Of the dark, being left alone, traffic, strangers, large animals, crowds.

The remedies. Again, it is the Bach Flower Remedies that shine here, especially cherry plum and mimulus.

Cognitive symptoms. Difficulty in concentration, poor memory.

---

*Adapted from: Hamilton, M. "The Assessment of Anxiety States by Rating," *British Journal of Medical Psychology*, 32, 1959, pp. 50–55.

The remedies. The specifics suggested for stress management given in the following pages are indicated with the possible addition of ginkgo and rosemary to help with difficulty in concentration and poor memory. Basil essential oil can be used to aid concentration as an inhalation. A "brain tonic" tea can easily be made to increase memory and improve the ability to concentrate. Mix the following herbs and infuse 1 to 2 teaspoonfuls of the mixture in a cup of boiling water for ten to fifteen minutes. Drink three times a day:

- Rosemary, 1 part
- Yerba maté, 1 part
- Ginkgo leaves, 4 parts
- Gotu kola, 2 parts

Depressed mood. Loss of interest, depression, diurnal mood swings. Lack of pleasure in hobbies, early waking.

The remedies. In addition to the herbal suggestions that follow, the Bach Flower Remedies can be especially relevant. Consider gentian, gorse, mustard, olive, sweet chestnut, and wild rose.

General body sensations. Tinnitus, hot and cold flushes, prickling sensations, blurred vision, feelings of weakness.

The remedies. All of the relaxing nervines and relaxing exercises will ease this group of symptoms.

Respiratory symptoms. Pressure of constriction in chest, tightness of breath, feelings of choking, sighing.

The remedies. All of the relaxing nervines and relaxing exercises will ease this group of symptoms.

Genitourinary symptoms. Frequency in urination, suppressed menstrual periods, frigidity, premature ejaculation, impotence, urgency of urination, excessive bleeding during period, loss of erection.

The remedies. These symptoms can be treated with herbal medicines that are not directly relevant to the topic of stress management. This highlights the need for competent diagnosis to ensure appropriate treatment. See *Herbs for Women's Health* by Mary Bove, N.D., and Linda Costarella, N.D., and *Herbs for Men's Health* by CJ Puotinen (Keats Publishing).

Physiological symptoms. Tremor of hands, strained face, swallowing, sweating, furrowed brow, facial pallor, belching, eyelid twitching.

The remedies. All of the antispasmodics, relaxing nervines, and relaxing exercises will ease this group of symptoms.

Tension. Feelings of tension, inability to relax, easily moved to tears, feelings of restlessness, fatigue, startled response, trembling.

The remedies. Again, the relaxing nervines and relaxing exercises will help, but in addition, the essential oils of lavender and rose geranium are especially helpful. The Bach Flower Remedies hornbeam, olive, and rock rose should also be considered.

General somatic symptoms. Muscular aches and pains, muscular twitching, muscular stiffness, grinding teeth.

The remedies. Muscle-relaxing antispasmodics such as crampbark and the stronger relaxing nervines such as valerian are effective here.

Cardiovascular symptoms. Tachycardia, chest pain, feelings of faintness, palpitations, throbbing of blood vessels, skipped heartbeats.

The remedies. Herbal medicine has much to offer for the

gentle treatment of heart problems in this body system and are discussed in *Herbs for the Heart* by CJ Puotinen (Keats Publishing).

Gastrointestinal symptoms. Difficulty in swallowing, indigestion, heartburn, looseness of bowels, constipation, gas, burps, bloating, weight loss.

The remedies. One of the strengths of herbal medicine is its efficacy in the treatment of digestive system problems, and especially those that are stress-related. This is discussed below and in much more depth in *Herbs to Improve Digestion* by CJ Puotinen (Keats Publishing).

Autonomic nervous system symptoms. Dry mouth, pallor, giddiness, flushing, tendency to sweat.

The remedies. All of the relaxing nervines and relaxing exercises will ease this group of symptoms.

Depression

Depression is a state of mind familiar to almost everyone, but this very familiarity becomes problematic when approaching clinical depressive states. In ordinary usage, the word refers to a mood state that in medicine is called *dysthymia*, as contrasted with the normal state of *euthymia* and the opposite state of elation. In psychiatric usage, disorders of mood are called affective disorders; depression can be such a disease in itself or a symptom of another mental disorder. Normal human responses to some situations may also include transient depressions.

Major depression occurs in 10 to 20 percent of the world's population in the course of a lifetime. Women are more often affected than men by a two-to-one ratio, and they seem to be at particular risk in the period prior to menstruation or following childbirth. Relatives of patients with major depression also seem to be at some higher risk of becoming depressed, and about 2 percent of the population may have a chronic disorder known as a depressive personality.

Depression is defined by a standard set of symptoms described in the American Psychiatric Association's *Diagnostic and Statistical Manual of Mental Disorders.* They are:

- Poor appetite and significant weight loss, or increased appetite and significant weight gain.
- Insomnia or increased sleep.
- Agitation or retardation of movement and thought.
- Loss of interest or pleasure in usual activities or decrease in sexual drive.
- Fatigue and loss of energy.
- Feelings of worthlessness, self-reproach, or excessive or inappropriate guilt.
- Diminished ability to think or concentrate; indecisiveness.
- Recurrent thoughts of death or suicide; or suicide attempts.

Not all of these characteristics occur in each individual who becomes depressed. For purposes of psychiatric treatment, a person is considered to have experienced a major depressive episode if he or she exhibits a loss of interest or pleasure in all or almost all usual activities and shows at least four of the above symptoms nearly every day for a period of at least two weeks. The term "depression" is often modified by words that imply either some specific factor, or some chemical mechanism is the cause of the state.

- Depressions that are reactions to some loss of or separation from a valued person or object are called reactive (or exogenous) depressions.

- This contrasts with the usually more severe depressions without apparent cause, called endogenous depressions, or those accompanied by delusions.

Specific Remedies for Depression

St. John's wort (*Hypericum*) has a long tradition of use in Europe, and while it sometimes gets remarkable results, it is also sometimes ineffective. It takes time to work, so it must be taken for at least a month.

A double-blind clinical trial was conducted in 1993 testing the antidepressant effects of St. John's wort extract. One hundred and five outpatients with depressions of short duration were treated in a double-blind study either with 300 mg of St. John's wort extract three times a day or with a placebo. After four weeks of treatment, 67 percent of the participants experienced a positive improvement.

Other lifestyle issues must also be addressed in the treatment of depression. From green salads to relaxation, from spinal adjustments to listening to music, the list is endless. Exercise is especially important. *The Textbook of Natural Medicine* by Joseph Pizzorno and Michael Murray, N.D., suggests the following nutritional supplements:

Basic Formula for Depression

- 2 parts St. John's wort
- 1 part oats
- 1 part lavender
- 1 part mugwort

Take 1 teaspoon of tincture three times a day for at least one month.

- Vitamin B complex, 50 to 150 mg daily
- Vitamin C, 1 gram three times daily
- Folic acid, 400 mcg daily
- Vitamin B$_{12}$, 250 mcg daily
- Magnesium, 500 mg daily

Indigestion

Digestive system symptoms can be an unpleasant way for the stress response to manifest.

Every herbalist and every culture have their favorite remedies for indigestion. European specifics include gentian, peppermint, chamomile, balm, hops, and valerian. Often a tea made from a single fresh remedy is best. This should be an herb with a taste and aroma. Ideally, it should be a plant you could easily cultivate, thus providing a steady supply of fresh leaves.

These simple teas can be augmented by using a combination of tinctures to aid the digestive system in general.

Hypertension

There are over 35 million hypertensives in the United States, with twice as many African-Americans as Caucasians. The reasons for this are

Indigestion Tincture

Mix equal parts:
- Gentian
- Chamomile
- Valerian
- Peppermint

Take ½ teaspoon ten minutes before eating.

not known. Although hypertension is a common problem in our culture, it is rare in cultures that are relatively untouched by the Western lifestyle. Stress plays a major role in causing and maintaining hypertension. Dietary, psychological, and social factors must all be addressed for any real change to occur.

Hypertension Formula

- 2 parts hawthorn
- 1 part linden
- 1 part yarrow
- 1 part crampbark
- 1 part valerian

Take 1 teaspoon of tincture three times a day.

Other plants might also be included depending upon the specific symptoms. Here is a possible mixture for hypertension where stress is a major factor.

- 2 parts hawthorn
- 1 part linden
- 1 part yarrow
- 1 part Siberian ginseng
- 1 part skullcap
- 1 part crampbark
- 1 part valerian

Take 1 teaspoon of tincture three times a day.

A number of herbs are specific for hypertension, usually working because of their impact on one or another of the processes involved in the condition's development. The most important plant remedy within Western medicine is hawthorn, probably followed by linden. Garlic is also effective for lowering high blood pressure and should be used in cooking and as a dietary supplement.

Premenstrual Syndrome (PMS)

This describes a broad range of symptoms that occur cyclically and which are severe enough to disturb a woman's life patterns or cause her to seek help from a health practitioner. Most women experience some body change cyclically during the menstruating years corresponding to the pattern of cycling hormones.

From my clinical experience, I would suggest skullcap as ideally suited for relief of the psychological symptoms, though various other remedies may act as well for specific women, so generalizations are problematic. Longer-term, hormonally focused herbal treatments are very effective but beyond the scope of this book.

The usual dosage of skullcap would be 1 heaped teaspoon of dried herb to 1 cup of boiling water, or ¼ teaspoon of the tincture, taken three times a day. This dosage may be increased until the desired relief is experienced. The dosage regime may be altered as necessary, varying time of day and quantity to suit individual needs. For example, one may take the whole dose first thing in the morning, or smaller amounts at frequent intervals throughout the day. The woman's experience is the guiding principle here.

Stress and Children

With its focus on preventive medicine, holistic approaches to health can be helpful in many of the common problems of childhood. If conditions are brought under control during childhood, they can often be avoided entirely in adult life. Children have special needs and special plants address these needs, but the most important consideration is the importance of tender loving care. Children respond to love and caring in wonderful ways. So do adults, if they give themselves the chance!

Children are susceptible to a variety of stresses, usually characterized by the feeling of being overwhelmed or threatened by more pressures and demands than they can handle. What constitutes a source of stress varies among children. One child may be stressed by changes in his daily routine, by moving to a new home, or by the birth of a sibling. These same events may strike another child as novel and enjoyable, and she may even thrive on such stimulation. Children also differ in their resilience and in how long it takes them to bounce back after stressful life events.

Coping usually requires thinking through the alternatives at hand and trying to make the best of stressful circumstances. However, a preschooler's capacity to analyze and formulate strategic plans is very limited. Getting help is therefore highly dependent upon an adult recognizing warning signs in youngsters struggling with stress. Once the problem is identified, the adult can help by listening to the child's expressions concerning stressful events and situations and offering understanding, support, reassurance, and abundant affection, holding, and cuddling. Coping with stress is easier when the child has a sense of self-esteem, which parents can and should

---

PROCEDURE: *Make an infusion using ½ to 1 teaspoon of the mixed herbs to 1 cup boiling water. Sweeten with honey. The dosage is 1 cup three times a day. Alternatively, add 10 drops of the mixed herbs in tincture form to a cup of juice.*

Nervine Tonics

- Oats
- St. John's wort
- Skullcap

Nervine Relaxants

- Hyssop
- Lavender
- Chamomile
- Balm
- Linden
- Red clover

Hypnotics

- California poppy
- Chamomile

Infant's Calming Herbal Bath

Here is a formulation created by Maribeth Riggs for overexcitability, anxiousness, or mild insomnia.

- 1 quart water
- 1 ounce dried lavender buds
- 1 ounce dried chamomile flowers

1. *Bring the water to a boil in a covered pot.*

2. *Remove the pot from the heat and add the herbs, being sure to cover the pot again. Let the herbs steep in the hot water for twenty minutes.*

3. *Strain and discard them. The bath tea is dark yellow and smells pleasantly of lavender.*

4. *Pour the tea into an infant bathtub and add enough warm water to fill it. The herbal bath should be as hot as a normal bath for the infant.*

APPLICATION: *Make sure the room is warm before the bath. Place the infant in the bathwater and hold him or her reassuringly, humming and crooning all the while. Soak the infant in the bath for at least ten minutes. Do not try to wash the infant during an herbal bath. Gently pour the water over the belly and legs and just let the infant play and splash. Use this bath as often as necessary to reassure and calm an upset, colicky infant.*

encourage, and when they have good verbal and problem-solving skills. Children also learn coping strategies by observing others around them. When adults exhibit calmness in the face of emergencies or other difficulties, children learn from this example and are less likely to pick up fears and are more likely to be able to cope with their own moments of difficulty.

A few of the many nervine remedies offered by nature are especially appropriate for problems of stress in children.

Hyperactivity

This is a thorny issue that raises a plethora of questions. There is no doubt that extreme hyperactivity occurs and can be related to dietary factors. This having been said, there is an unfortunate tendency for children to be labeled "hyperactive" simply because the teacher or parents do not have the patience for a very active, perceptive, inquisitive, or creative child.

The *Merck Manual* points out, quite rightly, that "claims that a child is hyperactive often reflect the tolerance level of the annoyed person." Since when has not fitting into the normal mold been a disease? The use of psychopharmaceuticals to control these children sounds a little bit like Soviet psychiatrists giving major tranquilizers to dissidents because they must (obviously) be insane to question the status quo. Rather than sedating our children so they can deal with their world, why not change the nature of schooling so it is more challenging and exciting?

Where the child is experiencing a real problem, there may be some help that can be provided herbally, provided that two areas are first addressed:

- **Psychological factors.**

- **Food irritants.** There is increasing evidence that food or chemical irritants play a significant role in hyper-activity. They may be pollutants (such as heavy metals) or artificial food additives (such as colorings or flavors).

For details and support with these two areas, contact The Feingold Association, 127 E. Main Street, Riverhead, NY 11901, (516) 369-9340.

Herbs to consider in supporting a broad treatment plan that also includes dietary and psychological aspects might be:

Chamomile	Milk thistle
Linden blossom	Red clover

These herbs can also help with stress and exhaustion in the parent! They may be used as teas or tinctures.

The following is a brief discussion of the herbs recommended for alleviating headaches, insomnia, and/or stress, showing their primary use and how to prepare and take them. A more detailed exploration of chamomile, kava kava, and valerian is given as an example of the depth in which clinicians must know their herbs.

ASHWAGANDHA   *Withania somnifera*

Part used	Root.
Actions	Adaptogen, sedative.
Indications	Ashwagandha is an herb from India used for the treatment of debility, impotence, and premature aging. Modern research has stressed its antitumor and adaptogenic actions, reinforcing its comparison with ginseng. However, ashwagandha occupies an important part in the herbal *materia medica*, because while it is not as potent as *Panax ginseng*, it lacks the stimulating effects of the latter. In fact, it has a mild sedative action as indicated by its specific name *somnifera*. This

makes it ideally suited to the treatment of overactive but debilitated people. Its indications include debility and nervous exhaustion especially due to stress, convalescence after acute illness, or extreme stress and chronic inflammatory diseases especially of connective tissue. It is ideally suited as a general tonic for disease prevention and for those under stress.

Preparation & dosage

INFUSION: Put ½ teaspoonful of the root in 1 cup of water, bring to a boil and simmer gently for 10 minutes. Drink 1 cup, 3 times a day. TINCTURE: Take ¼ to ½ teaspoon of the tincture 3 times a day.

BALM   *Melissa officinalis*

Part used

Dried aerial parts, or fresh in season.

Actions

Carminative, nervine, antispasmodic, diaphoretic, antimicrobial.

Indications

Balm is a relaxing, carminative herb that relieves spasms in the digestive tract and is often used in flatulent dyspepsia. It is especially helpful where there is dyspepsia associated with anxiety or depression, as the gently sedative oils relieve tension and anxiety reactions. It may also be used in migraine that is associated with tension, neuralgia, anxiety-induced palpitations, or insomnia. Extracts have antiviral properties and a lotion-based extract may be used for skin lesions of herpes simplex, the antiviral activity having been confirmed in both laboratory and clinical trials.

Preparation & dosage
INFUSION: Pour 1 cup of boiling water onto 1 to 2 teaspoonfuls of the dried herb or 4 to 6 fresh leaves and leave to infuse for 10 to 15 minutes, well covered. Take 1 cup of this tea in the morning and the evening, or when needed. TINCTURE: Take ¼ to ½ teaspoon of the tincture 3 times a day.

BLACK COHOSH   *Cimicifuga racemosa*

Part used
Root and rhizome; dried, not fresh.

Actions
Emmenagogue, antispasmodic, hypotensive, nervine.

Indications
Black cohosh offers a valuable combination of actions that makes it uniquely useful in painful cramping conditions of the female reproductive system. It may be used in cases of painful or delayed menstruation and ovarian cramps. It is also active in the treatment of rheumatic, muscular, and neurological pain. It is helpful in sciatica and neuralgia. As a relaxing nervine, it may be used in many situations where such an agent is needed. It has been found beneficial in cases of tinnitus.

Preparation & dosage
DECOCTION: Pour 1 cup of water onto ½ to 1 teaspoonful of the dried root and bring to a boil. Let it simmer for 10 to 15 minutes. Drink 1 cup 3 times a day. TINCTURE: Take ¼ to ½ teaspoon of the tincture 3 times a day.

BLACK HAW   *Viburnum prunifolium*

Part used	Dried bark of root, stem, or trunk.
Actions	Antispasmodic, hypotensive, astringent.
Indications	Black haw has very similar use to crampbark, to which it is closely related. It is an effective relaxant of the uterus and is used for dysmenorrhea and false labor pains as well as in threatened miscarriage. Its relaxant and sedative actions might explain its power in reducing blood pressure in hypertension, which happens through a relaxation of the peripheral blood vessels. It may be used as an antispasmodic in the treatment of asthma.
Preparation & dosage	DECOCTION: Put 2 teaspoonfuls of the dried bark in 1 cup of water, bring to a boil and simmer for 10 minutes. Drink 1 cup 3 times a day. TINCTURE: Take ½ to 1 teaspoon of the tincture 3 times a day.

BONESET   *Eupatorium perfoliatum*

Part used	Dried aerial parts.
Actions	Diaphoretic, bitter, laxative, tonic, antispasmodic, carminative, astringent.
Indications	Boneset is one of the best remedies for the relief of the associated symptoms that accompany influenza. It will speedily relieve the aches and pains as well as aid the body in dealing with any fever that is present. Boneset may also be used to help clear the upper respi-

ratory tract of mucus congestion. Its mild aperient activity will ease constipation. It may safely be used in any fever and also as a general cleansing agent. It may provide symptomatic aid in the treatment of muscular rheumatism.

Combinations In the treatment of influenza it may be combined with yarrow, elder flowers, cayenne, or ginger, and with pleurisy root and elecampane in bronchial conditions.

Preparation INFUSION: Pour 1 cup of boiling water onto 1
& dosage to 2 teaspoons of the dried herb and leave to infuse for 10 to 15 minutes. This should be taken as hot as possible. During fevers or the flu it should be taken every half hour. TINCTURE: Take ½ teaspoon of the tincture 3 times a day.

CALIFORNIA POPPY   *Eschscholtzia californica*

Part used Dried aerial parts.

Actions Nervine, hypnotic, antispasmodic, anodyne.

Indications A good general relaxing herb, it has been used as a sedative and hypnotic for children when there is overexcitability and sleeplessness. It can be used whenever an antispasmodic remedy is required.

Preparation INFUSION: Pour a cup of boiling water onto 1
& dosage to 2 teaspoonfuls of the dried herb and leave to infuse for 10 minutes. Drink a cup at night

to promote restful sleep. TINCTURE: Take ¼ to ¾ teaspoon of the tincture at night.

CELERY SEED   *Apium graveolens*

Part used   Dried ripe fruits.

Actions   Antirheumatic, anti-inflammatory, diuretic, carminative, antispasmodic, nervine.

Indications   Celery seeds are most useful as a component in the treatment of rheumatism, arthritis, and gout. They are especially helpful in rheumatoid arthritis where there is associated anxiety and mild depression. Their diuretic action is involved in rheumatic conditions, but they are also used as a urinary antiseptic, largely because of the volatile oil *apiol*.

Preparation   INFUSION: Pour 1 cup of boiling water onto 1
& dosage   to 2 teaspoons of freshly crushed seeds. Leave to infuse for 10 to 15 minutes. Drink 3 times a day. TINCTURE: Take 2 to 4 ml 3 times a day.

CHAMOMILE   *Matricaria recutita*

Part used   Flowering tops.

Actions   Nervine, antispasmodic, carminative, anti-inflammatory, antimicrobial, bitter, vulnerary.

Indications   A comprehensive list of chamomile's medical uses would be very long. Included would be insomnia, anxiety, menopausal depression, loss of appetite, dyspepsia, diarrhea, colic, aches and pains of the flu, migraine, neuralgia, teething, vertigo, motion sickness, conjunctivitis, inflamed skin, urticaria, and more. This may seem too good to be true, but it reflects the wide range of actions in the body.

Chamomile is probably the most widely used relaxing nervine herb in the Western world. It relaxes and tones the nervous system and is especially valuable where anxiety and tension produce digestive symptoms such as gas, colic pains, or even ulcers. This ability to focus on physical symptoms as well as underlying psychological tension is one of the great benefits of herbal remedies in stress and anxiety-related problems. It makes a wonderful late-night tea to ensure restful sleep. It is helpful with anxious children or teething infants, where it can be added to the bath.

As an antispasmodic herb, it works on the peripheral nerves and muscles so it indirectly relaxes the whole body. When the physical body is at ease, ease in the mind and heart follows. It can prevent or ease cramps in the muscles, such as the legs or abdomen. As an essential oil added to a bath, it relaxes the body after a hard day while easing the cares and weight of a troubled heart and mind.

Being rich in essential oils, chamomile acts on the digestive system, promoting proper function. This usually involves soothing the walls of the intestines, easing gripping pains, and helping with the removal of gas. It is an effective anti-inflammatory remedy internally for the digestive and respiratory systems as well as externally on the skin. A cup of hot chamomile tea is a simple, effective way of relieving indigestion, calming inflammation such as gastritis, and helping prevent ulcer formation. Using the essential oil as a steam inhalation will allow the oils to reach inflamed mucous membranes in the sinuses and lungs.

Chamomile is a mild antimicrobial, helping the body to destroy or resist pathogenic microorganisms. Azulene, one of the components of the essential oil, is bactericidal to *Staphylococcus* and *Streptococcus* infections. The oil from 0.10 gram of flowers is enough to destroy three times the amount of Staphylococcal toxins in two hours.

As an anticatarrhal, chamomile helps the body remove excess mucus buildup in the sinus area. It may be used in head colds and allergy reactions such as hay fever. Mucus is not a problem in itself. It is an essential body product, but when too much is produced, it is usually in response to an infection, helping the body remove the problematic organism, or to help the body remove excess carbohydrate.

A review of recent scientific literature shows how much interest this venerable folk remedy is still receiving. Most of the clinical therapeutic research comes from Europe, reflecting the respect chamomile receives in the medical community there. Anti-inflammatory effects have been the main focus of research, being the official criteria for its inclusion in the pharmacopoeia. These properties explain the herb's value in a wide range of digestive and intestinal problems. Taken by mouth or used as an enema, it is particularly helpful in colitis and irritable bowel syndrome. A fascinating recent German study demonstrated the efficacy of chamomile on the healing of wounds caused by tattooing. A common problem with tattoos is a "weeping" wound where the skin has been abraded. The healing and drying process was compared between patients who were treated with chamomile and a similar group who were not. The decrease of the weeping wound area as well as the speed of drying were dramatically improved in those using chamomile.

Clinical and laboratory research demonstrate statistically what the herbalist knows experientially, that chamomile will reduce inflammation and colic pain and protect against ulcer formation in the whole of the digestive tract.

Preparation & dosage

Chamomile may be used in all the ways plants can be prepared as medicines. Used fresh or dried it can be infused to make a tea. The tincture is an excellent way of ensuring all the plant's components are extracted and available for the body. In aromatherapy the essential oil of chamomile is a valued preparation. INFUSION: Pour a cup of boiling water over 2 to 3 teaspoons of fresh or dried herb and infuse for 10 minutes; drink 3 to 4 times a day. TINCTURE: Take 1 to 4 ml 3 times a day.

CRAMPBARK   *Viburnum opulus*

Part used   Dried bark.

Actions   Antispasmodic, anti-inflammatory, nervine, hypotensive, astringent.

Indications   Crampbark shows by its name the richly deserved reputation it has as a relaxer of muscular tension and spasm. It has two main areas of use, in muscular cramps and in ovarian and uterine muscle problems. Crampbark will relax the uterus and so relieve painful cramps associated with periods (dysmenorrhea). In a similar way, it may be used to protect from threatened miscarriage. Its astringent action gives it a role in the treatment of excessive blood loss in menstrual periods as well as bleeding associated with menopause.

Preparation   DECOCTION: Put 2 teaspoons of the dried
& dosage   bark into 1 cup of water and bring to the boil. Simmer gently for 10 to 15 minutes. Drink hot 3 times a day. TINCTURE: Take 4 to 8 ml of the tincture 3 times a day.

DAMIANA   *Turnera diffusa*

Part used   Dried leaves and stems.

Actions   Nerve tonic, antidepressant, urinary antisep-
                tic, laxative.

Indications   Damiana is a tonic-strengthening remedy for
                the nervous system in debilitated people. It
                has an ancient reputation as an aphrodisiac.
                While this may or may not be true, it has a
                definite tonic action on the central nervous
                and endocrine systems. As a useful antidepres-
                sant, damiana is considered to be a specific in
                cases of anxiety and depression where there is
                a sexual factor. It may be used to strengthen
                the male sexual system.

Preparation   INFUSION: Pour 1 cup of boiling water onto 1
& dosage   teaspoon of the dried leaves and let infuse for
                10 to 15 minutes. Drink 3 times a day.
                TINCTURE: Take 1 to 2 ml of the tincture 3
                times a day.

ECHINACEA   *Echinacea* spp.

Part used   Root.

Actions   Antimicrobial, immunomodulator, antica-
                tarrhal, alterative.

Indications   Echinacea is one of the primary remedies for
                helping the body rid itself of microbial
                infections. It is often effective against both
                bacterial and viral attacks, and may be used
                in conditions such as boils, septicemia, and

similar infections. In conjunction with other herbs, it may be used for any infection anywhere in the body. For example, in combination with yarrow or bearberry it will effectively stop cystitis. It is especially useful for infections of the upper respiratory tract such as laryngitis and tonsillitis, and for catarrhal conditions of the nose and sinus. In general, it may be used widely and safely. The tincture or decoction may be used as a mouthwash in the treatment of pyorrhoea and gingivitis. It may also be used as an external lotion to help septic sores and cuts.

Preparation & dosage
DECOCTION: Put 1 to 2 teaspoons of the roots in 1 cup of water and bring it slowly to boil. Let it simmer for 10 to 15 minutes. Strain. Drink 3 times a day. TINCTURE: Take ¼ to ½ teaspoon 3 times a day.

ELDER *Sambuscus nigra*

Part used
Bark, flowers, berries, leaves.

Actions
BARK: Purgative, emetic, diuretic. LEAVES: Externally emollient and vulnerary, internally as purgative, expectorant, diuretic, and diaphoretic. FLOWERS: Diaphoretic, anticatarrhal, antispasmodic. BERRIES: Diaphoretic, diuretic, laxative.

Indications
The elder tree is a medicine chest by itself! The leaves are used for bruises, sprains, wounds, and chilblains. It has been reported

that elder leaves may be useful in an ointment for tumors. Elder flowers are ideal for the treatment of colds and influenza. They are indicated in any catarrhal inflammation of the upper respiratory tract such as hay fever and sinusitis. Catarrhal deafness responds well to elder flowers. Elderberries have similar properties to the flowers with the addition of their usefulness in rheumatism.

Combinations　For colds and fevers, it may be used with peppermint, yarrow, or hyssop. For influenza combine it with boneset. For catarrhal states mix it with goldenrod.

Preparation & dosage　INFUSION: Pour 1 cup of boiling water onto 2 teaspoons of the dried or fresh blossoms and infuse for 10 minutes. Drink hot 3 times a day. JUICE: Boil fresh berries in water for 2 to 3 minutes, then express the juice. To preserve, bring to the boil with 1 part honey to 10 parts of juice. Take 1 cup diluted with hot water twice a day. OINTMENT: Take 3 parts of fresh elder leaves and heat them with 6 parts of melted petroleum jelly until the leaves are crisp. Strain and store. TINCTURE: Take ¼ teaspoon of the tincture (made from the flowers) 3 times a day.

EYEBRIGHT　　　　　　　　　　*Euphrasia officinalis*

Part used　Dried aerial parts.

Actions　Anticatarrhal, astringent, anti-inflammatory.

Indications   Eyebright is an excellent remedy for the problems of mucous membranes. The combination of anti-inflammatory and astringent properties make it relevant in many conditions. Used internally, it is a powerful anticatarrhal and thus may be used to treat nasal catarrh, sinusitis, and other congestive states. It is best known for its use in conditions of the eye, where it is helpful in acute or chronic inflammations, stinging and weeping eyes, as well as oversensitivity to light. Used as a compress externally in conjunction with internal use, it is valuable in conjunctivitis and blepharitis.

Combinations   In catarrhal conditions, it combines well with goldenrod, elder flower, or goldenseal. In allergic conditions where the eyes are affected, it may be combined with ephedra. As an eye lotion, it may be mixed with goldenseal and distilled witch hazel.

Preparation & dosage   INFUSION: Pour a cup of boiling water onto 1 teaspoon of the dried herb and leave to infuse for 5 to 10 minutes. Strain. Drink 3 times a day. COMPRESS: Place 1 teaspoon of the dried herb in 1 pint of water and boil for 10 minutes, let cool slightly and strain. Moisten a compress (cotton wool, gauze, or muslin) in the lukewarm liquid, wring out slightly, and place over the eyes. Leave the compress in place for 15 minutes. Repeat several times a day. TINCTURE: Take ¼ teaspoon 3 times a day.

FEVERFEW   *Tanacetum parthenium*

Part used	Leaves.
Actions	Anti-inflammatory, vasodilator, emmenagogue, bitter.
Indications	Feverfew has regained its deserved reputation as a primary remedy in the treatment of migraine headaches, especially those that are relieved by applying warmth to the head. It may also help arthritis in the painfully active inflammatory stage. Dizziness and tinnitus may be eased, especially if it is used in conjunction with other remedies. Painful periods and sluggish menstrual flow will be relieved by feverfew. It is the only herb used in European phytotherapy known to be specific for the treatment of migraine. It is also the best example of a remedy well known to medical herbalists that has recently been accepted and used by allopathic medicine. It has been used throughout recorded medical history as a bitter tonic and remedy for severe headaches.
Preparation & dosage	It is best to use the equivalent of one fresh leaf 1 to 3 times a day. Preferably use fresh, but tincture or tablets are adequate. In this case, freeze-dried leaf preparations will be best (50 to 100 mg a day).

GINKGO   *Ginkgo biloba*

Part used	Leaves.
Actions	Anti-inflammatory, vasodilator.

Indications   Recent research has confirmed ginkgo's profound activity on brain function and cerebral circulation, and clinically it is proving effective in a range of vascular disorders, especially those due to restricted cerebral blood flow, and milder problems of normal aging such as weak memory, poor concentration, and depression. Ginkgo has been suggested for a wide range of conditions: vertigo, tinnitus, inner ear disturbances including partial deafness, impairment of memory and ability to concentrate, diminished intellectual capacity and alertness as a result of insufficient circulation, dementia, Alzheimer's disease, complications of stroke and skull injuries, diminished sight and hearing ability due to vascular insufficiency, intermittent claudication as a result of arterial obstruction, Raynaud's disease, and cerebral vascular and nutritional insufficiency.

Preparation   Ginkgo is becoming available in a number
& dosage   of different forms. The daily dose used in most studies is 27 mg of ginkgo glycosides, which corresponds to 6 to 12 grams of leaf, depending on the quality of the leaf. Products are usually standardized to contain 24 percent flavone glycosides and hence are highly concentrated compared to the original leaf. It is recommended at a dose of 120 mg daily in two to three divided doses.

GINGER
Zingiber officinale

Part used   Rootstock.

Actions   Stimulant, carminative, antispasmodic, rubefacient, diaphoretic, emmenagogue.

Indications   Ginger may be used as a stimulant of the peripheral circulation in cases of circulation, chilblains, and cramps. In feverish conditions, ginger acts as a useful diaphoretic, promoting perspiration. As a gargle it may be effective in the relief of sore throats. Externally it is the basis of many fibrositis and muscle sprain treatments. Ginger has been used worldwide as an aromatic carminative and pungent appetite stimulant. In India, and in other countries with hot and humid climates, ginger is eaten daily and is a well-known remedy for digestion problems. Its widespread use is not only due to its lively flavor but to its antioxidant and antimicrobial effects, necessary for the preservation of food, which is essential in such climates.

Preparation & dosage   INFUSION: Pour 1 cup of boiling water onto 1 teaspoon of the fresh root and let it infuse for 5 minutes. Drink whenever needed. DECOCTION: If you are using the dried root in powdered or finely chopped form, make a decoction by putting 1½ teaspoons in 1 cup of water. Bring it to a boil and simmer for 5 to 10 minutes. Drink whenever needed.

GINSENG, KOREAN AND AMERICAN   *Panax* spp.

Habitat   *Panax ginseng* is native to China and culti-
                   vated extensively in China, Korea, Japan, and
                   Russia. *Panax quinquefolia* is native to North
                   America.

Part used   Root.

Actions   Adaptogen, tonic, stimulant, hypoglycemic.

Indications   Ginseng has an ancient history and as such
                   has accumulated much folklore about its
                   actions and uses. The genus name *Panax*
                   derives from the Latin *panacea* meaning "cure
                   all." Many of the claims that surround it are,
                   unfortunately, exaggerated, but it is clear that
                   this is an important remedy. A powerful
                   adaptogen, it has a wide range of possible
                   therapeutic uses. The best therapeutic applica-
                   tion is with weak or elderly people, where the
                   adaptogenic and stimulating properties can be
                   profoundly useful. It should not be used
                   indiscriminately as the stimulating properties
                   can be contraindicated in some pathologies;
                   for example, Chinese herbalism warns against
                   ginseng being used in acute inflammatory
                   disease and bronchitis.

Preparation   Put ½ to 1 teaspoon of the root in 1 cup of
& dosage   water, bring to a boil and simmer gently for
                   10 minutes. Drink 3 times a day. TINCTURE:
                   Take 1 to 2 ml of the tincture 3 times a day
                   for up to 3 months.

GOLDENROD   *Solidago virgaurea*

Part used	Dried aerial parts.
Actions	Anticatarrhal, anti-inflammatory, antimicrobial, astringent, diaphoretic, carminative, diuretic.
Indications	Goldenrod is perhaps the first plant to think of for upper respiratory catarrh, whether acute of chronic; it may be used in combination with other herbs in the treatment of influenza. The carminative properties reveal a role in the treatment of flatulent dyspepsia. As an anti-inflammatory urinary antiseptic, Goldenrod may be use in cystitis, urethritis, and the like. It can be used to promote the healing of wounds. As a gargle, it can be used in laryngitis and pharyngitis.
Combinations	For upper respiratory catarrh, it may be used with eyebright, elder, echinacea, poke root, and wild indigo.
Preparation & dosage	INFUSION: Pour 1 cup of boiling water onto 2 to 3 teaspoons of the dried herb and leave to infuse for 10 to 15 minutes. Strain and drink 3 times a day. TINCTURE: Take ½ teaspoon 3 times a day.

HOPS   *Humulus lupulus*

Part used	Flower inflorescence.
Actions	Sedative, hypnotic, antimicrobial, antispasmodic, astringent.

Indications Hops is a remedy that has a marked relaxing effect upon the central nervous system. It is used extensively for the treatment of insomnia. It will ease tension and anxiety, and may be used where this tension leads to restlessness, headache, and possibly indigestion. As an astringent, with these relaxing properties it can be used in conditions such as colitis. It should, however, be avoided where there is a marked degree of depression as this may be accentuated. Externally, the antiseptic action is utilized for the treatment of ulcer. CAUTION: Do not use in cases of acute depression.

Preparation & dosage INFUSION: Pour 1 cup of boiling water onto 1 teaspoon of the dried flowers and let infuse for 10 to 15 minutes. Drink 1 cup before bed to induce sleep. This dose may be strengthened if needed. TINCTURE: Take 1 to 2 ml of the tincture 3 times a day.

HYSSOP   *Hyssopus officinalis*

Part used Dried aerial parts.

Actions Antispasmodic, expectorant, diaphoretic, nervine, anti-inflammatory, carminative.

Indications Hyssop has an interesting range of uses that are largely attributable to the antispasmodic action of the volatile oil. It is used in coughs, bronchitis, and chronic catarrh. Its diaphoretic properties explain its use in the common cold.

As a nervine it may be used in anxiety states, hysteria, and petit mal (a form of epilepsy).

Preparation & dosage

INFUSION: Pour 1 cup of boiling water onto 1 to 2 teaspoons of the dried herb and leave to infuse for 10 to 15 minutes. Drink 3 times a day. TINCTURE: Take 1 to 2 ml of the tincture 3 times a day.

KAVA KAVA *Piper methysticum*

Part used

Rhizome.

Actions

Relaxing nervine, hypnotic, antispasmodic, local anesthetic, antifungal.

Indications

Kava kava is a safe treatment for anxiety problems as at normal therapeutic doses it does not reduce alertness or interact with mild alcohol consumption. Unlike the benzodiazepine drugs, e.g., Valium, there is no risk of tolerance or addiction with kava. Its slight antidepressant activity makes it particularly suitable for the treatment of anxiety associated with minor forms of depression. Kava kava is one of the more effective and safe relaxants of skeletal muscle known in the plant kingdom. This property makes it useful for the treatment of nervous tension and conditions associated with skeletal muscle spasm and tension, such as headaches due to neck tension. Although pharmacological tests indicate that kava kava is not a sedative in the same sense as the benzodiazepines, it is an excellent hypnotic for the treatment of mild insomnia. High doses of kava kava do cause marked sedation, but such doses are not relevant to normal clinical use. A mild anticonvulsant action of kava may be useful in the treatment of epilepsy, but kava kava is not sufficiently active to control this condition on its own. The local anesthetic action on mucous membranes makes it useful for pain control in oral conditions. Kava kava douches have been successfully used for vaginal itching. Kava kava is also active as a topical antifungal agent.

Preparation & dosage

DECOCTION: Put 1 to 2 teaspoons of the rhizome in 1 cup of water, bring to boil and simmer gently for 10 to 15 minutes; drink as needed. TINCTURE: Take 3 to 6 ml per day. Standardized preparations should supply 100 to 200 mg of kava lactones per day. Long-term use of a dose equivalent to 400 mg or more of kava lactones per day may cause a scaly skin rash in some people.

KOLA   *Cola vera*

Part used

Seed kernel.

Actions

Stimulant to central nervous system, antidepressive, astringent, diuretic.

Indications

Kola has a marked stimulating effect on human consciousness. It can be used wherever there is a need for direct stimulation, which is less often than is usually thought, since, with good health and therefore right functioning, the nervous system does not need such help. In the short term, it may be used in nervous debility and in states of atony and weakness. It can act as a specific in nervous diarrhea. It will aid in states of depression and may, in some people, give rise to euphoric states. In some varieties of migraine it can help greatly. It can be viewed as a specific in cases of depression associated with weakness and debility.

Preparation & dosage

DECOCTION: Put 1 to 2 teaspoons of the powdered nuts in a cup of water, bring to boil and simmer gently for 10 to 15 minutes. Drink when needed. TINCTURE: Take ¼ to ½ teaspoon of the tincture 3 times a day.

LAVENDER   *Lavandula officinalis*

Part used

Flowers.

Actions

Carminative, antispasmodic, antidepressant, emmenagogue, hypotensive.

Indications

This beautiful herb has many uses—culinary, cosmetic, and medicinal. It is often an effective herb for headaches, especially when they are related to stress. Lavender can be quite effective in the clearing of depression, especially if used in conjunction with other remedies. As a gentle strengthening tonic of the nervous system, it may be used in states of nervous debility and exhaustion. It can be used to soothe and promote natural sleep. Externally, the oil may be used as a stimulating liniment to help ease the aches and pains of rheumatism.

Preparation & dosage

INFUSION: To take internally, pour 1 cup of boiling water onto 1 teaspoon of the dried herb and leave to infuse for 10 minutes. Drink 3 times a day. EXTERNAL USE: The oil should not be taken internally but can be inhaled, rubbed on the skin, or used in baths.

LEMON BALM   *Melissa officinalis*

Part used

Dried aerial parts or fresh in season.

Actions

Carminative, nervine, antispasmodic, diaphoretic, antimicrobial.

Indications

Balm is a relaxing, carminative herb that relieves spasms in the digestive tract and is often used in flatulent dyspepsia. It is especially helpful where there is dyspepsia associated with anxiety or depression, as the gently sedative oils relieve tension and anxiety reactions. It may also be used in migraine that is associated with tension, neuralgia, anxiety-induced palpitations, or insomnia. Extracts have antiviral properties, and a lotion-based extract may be used for skin lesions of herpes simplex, the antiviral activity having been confirmed both in laboratory and clinical trials.

Preparation & dosage

INFUSION: Pour 1 cup of boiling water onto 1 to 2 teaspoons of the dried herb or 4 to 6 fresh leaves and leave to infuse for 10 to 15 minutes, well covered. A cup of this tea should be taken in the morning and the evening or when needed. TINCTURE: Take 1 to 2 ml of the tincture 3 times a day.

LINDEN   *Tilia europea*

Part used Dried flowers.

Actions Nervine, antispasmodic, hypotensive, diaphoretic, diuretic, anti-inflammatory, astringent.

Indications Linden is well known as a relaxing remedy for use in nervous tension. It has a reputation as a prophylactic against the development of arteriosclerosis and hypertension. It is considered a specific in the treatment of raised blood pressure associated with arteriosclerosis and nervous tension. Its relaxing action combined with a general effect upon the circulatory system gives linden a role in the treatment of some forms of migraine. The diaphoresis combined with the relaxation explain its value in feverish colds and flu.

Preparation & dosage INFUSION: Pour 1 cup of boiling water onto 1 teaspoon of the blossoms and leave to infuse for 10 minutes. Drink 3 times a day. For a diaphoretic effect in fever, use 2 to 3 teaspoons. TINCTURE: Take 1 to 2 ml of the tincture 3 times a day.

MEADOWSWEET   *Filipendula ulmaria*

Part used	Aerial parts.
Actions	Antirheumatic, anti-inflammatory, carminative, antacid, antiemetic, astringent.
Indications	Meadowsweet is one of the best digestive remedies available and as such is indicated in many conditions if they are approached holistically. It acts to protect and soothe the mucous membranes of the digestive tract, reducing excess acidity and easing nausea. It is used in the treatment of heartburn, hyperacidity, gastritis, and peptic ulceration. Its gentle astringency is useful in treating diarrhea in children. The presence of aspirinlike chemicals explains meadowsweet's action in reducing fever and relieving the pain of rheumatism in muscles and joints.
Combinations	With marshmallow and chamomile, it is very soothing for a whole range of digestive problems. For musculoskeletal conditions, consider combining with black cohosh, willow bark, and celery seed for its anti-inflammatory effects.
Preparation & dosage	INFUSION: Pour 1 cup of boiling water over 1 to 2 teaspoons of the dried herb and leave to infuse for 10 to 15 minutes. Strain and drink 3 times a day or as needed. TINCTURE: Take ¼ to ½ teaspoon 3 times a day.

MOTHERWORT   *Leonurus cardiaca*

Part used	Aerial parts.
Actions	Nervine, emmenagogue, antispasmodic, cardiac tonic, hypotensive.
Indications	The names of this plant show its range of uses. *Motherwort* indicates its relevance to menstrual and uterine conditions while *cardiaca* indicates its use in heart and circulation treatments. It is valuable in the stimulation of delayed or suppressed menstruation, especially where there is anxiety or tension involved. It is a useful relaxing tonic for aiding in menopausal changes. It may be used to ease false labor pains. It is an excellent tonic for the heart, strengthening without straining. It is considered to be a specific in cases of tachycardia (heart palpitations), especially when brought about by anxiety and other such causes. It may be used in all heart conditions that are associated with anxiety and tension.
Preparation & dosage	INFUSION: Pour 1 cup of boiling water onto 1 to 2 teaspoons of the dried herb and leave to infuse for 10 to 15 minutes. Drink 3 times a day. TINCTURE: Take 1 to 4 ml of the tincture 3 times a day.

MUGWORT   *Artemisia vulgaris*

Part used	Leaves or root.
Actions	Bitter tonic, nervine tonic, emmenagogue.

Indications   Mugwort can be used whenever a digestive stimulant is called for. It will aid the digestion through the bitter stimulation of the juices while also providing a carminative oil. It has a mildly nervine action in aiding depression and easing tension, which appears to be due to the volatile oil, so it is essential that this is not lost in preparation. Mugwort may also be used as an emmenagogue in the aiding of normal menstrual flow.

Preparation & dosage   INFUSION: Pour 1 cup of boiling water onto 1 to 2 teaspoons of the dried herb and leave to infuse for 10 to 15 minutes in a covered container. Drink 3 times a day. Mugwort is used as a flavoring in a number of aperitif drinks, such as vermouth—a pleasant way to take it! TINCTURE: Take 1 to 2 ml of the tincture 3 times a day.

OATSTRAW   *Avena sativa*

Part used   Seeds and whole plant.

Actions   Nervine tonic, antidepressant, nutritive, demulcent, vulnerary.

Indications   Oatstraw is one of the best remedies for nourishing the nervous system, especially when under stress. It is considered a specific in cases of nervous debility and exhaustion when associated with depression. It may be used with most of the other nervines, both relaxant and stimulatory, to strengthen the whole of the nervous system. It is also used in general debility.

Preparation & dosage

INFUSION: Pour 1 cup of boiling water onto 1 to 3 teaspoons of the dried oatstraw and leave to infuse 10 to 15 minutes. Drink 3 times a day. TINCTURE: Take 3 to 5 ml 3 times a day. BATH: A soothing bath for use in neuralgia and irritated skin conditions can be made as follows. Boil 1 pound of shredded oatstraw in 2 quarts of water for ½ hour. Strain the liquid and add to the bath; alternatively, put cooked rolled oats into a muslin bag and use it to bathe with.

PASSIONFLOWER *Passiflora incarnata*

Part used

Leaves and whole plant.

Actions

Nervine, hypnotic, antispasmodic, anodyne, hypotensive.

Indications

Passionflower has a depressant effect on central nervous system activity and is hypotensive; thus it is used for its sedative and soothing properties to lower blood pressure and for insomnia. The alkaloids and flavonoids have both been reported to have sedative activity in animals. Many of the flavonoids, such as *apigenin*, are well-known for pharmacological activity, particularly antispasmodic and anti-inflammatory activities. It is the herb of choice for treating intransigent insomnia. It aids the transition into a restful sleep without any narcotic hangover. It may be used wherever an antispasmodic is required, e.g., in Parkinson's disease, seizures, and hysteria. It can help in relieving nerve pain such as neuralgia and the viral infection of nerves called shingles.

Preparation & dosage

INFUSION: Pour 1 cup of boiling water onto 1 to 2 teaspoons of the dried herb and let infuse for 15 minutes. Drink 1 cup in the evening for sleeplessness and 1 cup 2 times a day for the easing of other conditions. TINCTURE: Take 1 to 4 ml of the tincture and use in the same way as the infusion.

PRICKLY ASH   *Zanthoxylum americanum*

Part used

Bark and berries.

Actions

Stimulant (circulatory), tonic, alterative, carminative, diaphoretic, antirheumatic, hepatic.

Indications

Prickly ash may be used in a way that is similar to cayenne, although it is slower in action. It is used in many chronic problems such as rheumatism and skin diseases. Any sign of poor circulation calls for the use of this herb, such as chilblains, leg cramps, varicose veins, and varicose ulcers. Externally, it may be used as a stimulating liniment for rheumatism and fibrositis. Due to its stimulating effect on the lymphatic system, circulation, and mucous membranes, it has a role in the holistic treatment of many specific conditions.

Preparation & dosage

INFUSION: Pour 1 cup of boiling water onto 1 to 2 teaspoons of the bark and let infuse for 10 to 15 minutes. Strain and drink 3 times a day. TINCTURE: Take ¼ to ½ teaspoon 3 times a day.

PULSATILLA   *Anemone pulsatilla*

Part used

Aerial parts.

Actions

Nervine, antispasmodic, antibacterial.

Indications

Pulsatilla is an effective relaxing nervine for use in problems relating to nervous tension and spasm in the reproductive system. It may be used with safety in the relief of painful periods, ovarian pain, and painful conditions of the testes. It may be used to reduce tension reactions and headache associated with them. It will help insomnia and general overactivity. The antibacterial actions give this herb a role in treating infections that affect the skin, especially boils. It is similarly useful in the treatment of respiratory infections and asthma. The oil or tincture will ease earache.

Preparation & dosage

INFUSION: Pour 1 cup of boiling water onto ½ teaspoon of the dried herb and leave to infuse for 10 to 15 minutes. Drink 3 times a day or when needed. TINCTURE: Take ½ to 1 ml 3 times a day.

RED CLOVER   *Trifolium pratense*

Part used	Flower heads.
Actions	Alterative, expectorant, antispasmodic.
Indications	As a gentle, relaxing nervine, red clover has a unique use as a safe and gentle sedative for hyperactive children. It is one of the most useful remedies for children with skin problems. It may be used with complete safety in any case of childhood eczema. It may also be of value in other chronic skin conditions such as psoriasis. While most useful with children, it can also be of value for adults. The expectorant and antispasmodic action give this remedy a role in the treatment of coughs and bronchitis, especially in whooping cough. As an alterative it is indicated in a wide range of problems when used in a holistic sense.
Preparation & dosage	INFUSION: Pour 1 cup of boiling water onto 1 to 4 teaspoons of the dried herb and leave to infuse for 10 to 15 minutes. Drink 3 times a day. TINCTURE: Take 2 to 4 ml of the tincture 3 times a day.

SIBERIAN GINSENG   *Eleutherococcus senticosus*

Part used	Root.
Actions	Adaptogen.
Indications	Siberian ginseng can be recommended as a general tonic with a very wide range of clinical indications because of its nonspecific

action. It is especially useful in conditions impacted by the stress response, including angina, hypertension, hypotension, various types of neuroses, chronic bronchitis, and cancer. It can also be used to treat the effects of prolonged stress or overwork such as exhaustion, irritability, insomnia, and mild depression. Siberian ginseng can also assist in the recovery from acute or chronic diseases, trauma, surgery, and other stressful episodes, as well as counter the debilitating effects of chronic disease and treatments such as chemotherapy, radiation, and surgery. It can be taken on a long-term basis to minimize the incidence of acute infections and to generally improve well-being.

Preparation & dosage   The standard dosage of the tincture, based on clinical studies, is 2 to 4 ml 3 times a day. An equivalent dosage in capsule form, using a solid extract concentrated at a ratio of 20:1, would be 100 to 200 mg. The recommended regime is usually for a 6-week course followed by a 2-week break. This regime can be repeated for as long as necessary.

SKULLCAP   *Scutellaria laterifolia*

Part used   Aerial parts.

Actions   Nervine tonic, antispasmodic, hypotensive.

Indications   Skullcap is perhaps the most widely relevant nervine available to us in the *materia medica*. It relaxes states of nervous tension while at the same time renewing and revivifying the central nervous system. It has a specific use in the treatment of seizure and hysterical states as well as epilepsy. It may be used in all exhausted or depressed conditions. It can be used with complete safety in the easing of premenstrual tension.

Preparation & dosage
INFUSION: Pour 1 cup of boiling water onto 1 to 2 teaspoons of the dried herb and leave to infuse for 10 to 15 minutes. Drink 3 times a day or when needed. TINCTURE: Take 2 to 4 ml of the tincture 3 times a day.

ST. JOHN'S WORT *Hypericum perforatum*

Part used
Aerial parts.

Actions
Anti-inflammatory, antidepressant, astringent, vulnerary, nervine, antimicrobial.

Indications
Taken internally, St. John's wort has a sedative and mild pain-reducing effect, which gives it a place in the treatment of neuralgia, anxiety, tension, and similar problems. It is especially regarded as an herb to use where there are menopausal changes triggering irritability and anxiety. It is increasingly recommended for the treatment of depression. The standardized extract is recognized by the German government as an effective treatment for depressive states, fear, and nervous disturbances. In addition to neuralgic pain, it will ease fibrositis, sciatica, and rheumatic pain.

Externally, it is a valuable healing and anti-inflammatory remedy. As a lotion it will speed the healing of wounds and bruises, varicose veins, and mild burns. The oil is especially useful for the healing of sunburn.

Preparation & dosage

INFUSION: Pour 1 cup of boiling water onto 1 to 2 teaspoons of the dried herb and leave to infuse for 10 to 15 minutes. Drink 3 times a day. TINCTURE: Take 1 to 4 ml of the tincture 3 times a day. CAPSULES: In the treatment of depression the recommended dose is 300 mg of concentrated dry extract standardized to 0.3% hypericin taken 3 times daily.

THYME   *Thymus vulgaris*

Part used

Leaves and flowering tops.

Actions

Carminative, antimicrobial, antispasmodic, expectorant, astringent, anthelmintic.

Indications

With its high content of volatile oil, thyme makes a good carminative for use in dyspepsia and sluggish digestion. This oil is also a strongly antiseptic substance, which explains many of its uses. It can be used externally as a lotion for infected wounds but also internally for respiratory and digestive infections. It may be used as a gargle in laryngitis and tonsillitis, easing sore throats and soothing irritable coughs. It is an excellent cough remedy, producing expectoration and reducing unnecessary spasm. It may be used in bronchitis, whooping cough, and asthma. A warm infusion is beneficial in headache and to promote perspiration.

Preparation & dosage

INFUSION: Pour 1 cup of boiling water onto 2 teaspoons of the dried herb and let infuse for 10 minutes. Strain and drink 3 times a day. TINCTURE: Take ½ teaspoon 3 times a day.

VALERIAN   *Valeriana officinalis*

Part used

Rhizome, stolons, and roots.

Actions

Nervine, hypnotic, antispasmodic, carminative, hypotensive.

Indications

Valerian has a wide range of specific uses, but its main indications are anxiety, nervous sleeplessness, and the bodily symptoms of tension such as muscle cramping or indigestion. It may be used safely in situations where tension and anxiety are causing problems. This may manifest in purely psychological and behavioral ways or with body symptoms. Valerian will help in most cases. For some people it can be an effective mild pain reliever.

As one of the best gentle and harmless herbal sleeping remedies, it enhances the natural body process of slipping into sleep and making the stresses of the day recede. For people who do not need as much sleep as they once did, it also eases lying awake in bed, ensuring that it becomes a restful and relaxing experience. This is often as revivifying as sleep itself, and indeed all that is necessary in many cases. The true nature of sleep still remains a mystery. Everybody goes through stages of REM (rapid eye movement) sleep, a stage where dreaming is associated with minor involuntary muscle jerks and rapid eye movements indicating that active processes are occurring in the brain. It is important not to suppress the dreams that occur during this stage. Emotional experiences are processed by the mind in those dreams, and events arising from both the unconscious and daily life are balanced and harmonized. While sleeping pills have a marked impact on REM sleep, valerian does not interfere with this process as it is not powerful enough to suppress the necessary REM phases.

The research into valerian confirms the traditional experience of the herbalist. One study found that patients who used valerian reported significant improvement in the quality of their sleep. Improvement was most notable among those smokers who considered themselves poor or irregular sleepers. Dream recall was relatively unaffected by valerian. When the effect of valerian root on sleep was studied in healthy young people, it was shown to reduce perceived sleep latency and decrease wake time after sleep onset. In other words, those studied experienced an easier and quicker descent into sleep. A combination of valerian and hops was given to people whose sleep was disturbed by heavy traffic noise. Giving the herbs well before retiring reduced the noise-induced disturbance of a number of sleep-stage patterns.

Much research has centered on valerian's effects upon smooth muscle, demonstrating that it is a powerful and safe muscle relaxant. It can be safely used in muscle cramping, uterine cramps, and intestinal colic. Its sedative and antispasmodic action can be partially ascribed to the *valepotriates* and to a lesser extent to the *sesquiterpene* constituents of the volatile oils. Among other effects, valerian decreases both spontaneous and caffeine-stimulated muscular activity, significantly reduces aggressiveness of animals, and decreases a number of measurable processes in the brain.

Italian researchers compared the relaxing properties of valerian and a number of other plants on the muscles of the digestive tract. Hawthorn and valerian were the most relaxing, followed by passionflower and chamomile. Especially interesting was the finding that combining all the herbs acted in a synergistic way, causing a relaxation response at low dosage levels.

Valerian is used worldwide as a relaxing remedy in hypertension and stress-related heart problems. There is an effect here beyond simple nerve relaxation, as valerian contains alkaloids that are mild hypotensives. Such use is recognized by the World Health

Organization (WHO), which promotes the research and development of traditional medicine and recognizes the importance of using whole plants, going beyond the test tube for meaningful results. In WHO-sponsored studies in Bulgaria, traditional herbs known for their healing effect in cardiovascular problems were studied and the results of the clinical examinations of patients using these herbs were impressive. Valerian was one herb whose use was validated. Others were garlic, geranium, European mistletoe, olive, and hawthorn.

A very small number of people experience what has been described as a paradoxical response to valerian. In other words, instead of the psychological and muscular relaxation expected, a form of stimulation occurs that is often experienced like drinking too much coffee. If this occurs, it is a transitory stimulation but probably means the person will always have this response to valerian and thus should avoid it. Passionflower provides a very appropriate alternative for sleeping difficulties, whereas skullcap is an appropriate daytime relaxing herb alternative.

Preparation & dosage

To be highly effective, valerian has to be used in sufficiently high dosage. The tincture is the most widely used preparation and is always useful, provided that the single dose is not counted in drops but rather that 2.5 to 5 ml (½ to 1 teaspoon) be given, and indeed sometimes 10 ml at one time. It is pointless to give 10 to 20 drops of valerian tincture. Overdosage is highly unlikely, even with very much larger doses. For situations of extreme stress where a sedative or muscle-relaxant effect is needed fast, the single dose of 1 teaspoon may be repeated 2 or 3 times at short intervals.

The dried herb can be prepared as an infusion to ensure no loss of the volatile oil. One to 2 teaspoons of the dried herb are used for each cup of tea prepared. With these doses, expect a good relaxing, antispasmodic, and sleep-inducing effect, and above all rapid sedation in states of excitement. A cold infusion may also be used; pour 1 glass of cold water over 1 to 2 teaspoons of valerian root and let stand 8 to 10 hours. A nighttime dose can thus be set up in the morning, and a dose for the mornings can be prepared at night.

VERVAIN   *Verbena officinalis*

Part used	Aerial parts.
Actions	Nervine tonic, sedative, antispasmodic, diaphoretic, hypotensive, galactagogue, hepatic.
Indications	Vervain is an herb that will strengthen the nervous system while relaxing any tension and stress. It can be used to ease depression and melancholia, especially when this follows illness such as influenza. Vervain may be used to help in seizure and hysteria. As a

diaphoretic, it can be used in the early stages of fevers. As a hepatic remedy it helps in inflammation of the gallbladder and jaundice. It may be used as a mouthwash against caries and gum disease.

Preparation & dosage

INFUSION: Pour 1 cup of boiling water onto 1 to 4 teaspoons of the dried herb and leave to infuse for 10 to 15 minutes. Drink 3 times a day. TINCTURE: Take 2 to 4 ml of the tincture 3 times a day.

VITEX (CHASTEBERRY) *Vitex agnus-castus*

Part used

Fruit.

Actions

Hormonal normalizer.

Indications

Vitex or chasteberry has the effect of stimulating and normalizing pituitary gland functions, especially the progesterone function. It may be called an amphoteric remedy, as it can produce apparently opposite effects, though in truth it is simply normalizing. It has, for instance, a reputation as both an aphrodisiac and an anaphrodisiac! It will usually enable what is appropriate to occur. The greatest use of vitex lies in normalizing the activity of female sex hormones and it is thus indicated for dysmenorrhea, premenstrual stress, and other disorders related to hormone function. It is especially beneficial during menopausal changes. In a similar way, it may be used to aid the body to regain a natural balance after the use of the birth control pill.

Preparation & dosage	INFUSION: Pour 1 cup boiling water onto 1 teaspoon of the ripe berries and leave to infuse for 10 to 15 minutes. Strain and drink 3 times a day. TINCTURE: Take ¼ teaspoon 3 times a day.

WHITE POPLAR *Populus tremuloides*

Part used	Bark.
Actions	Anti-inflammatory, astringent, antiseptic, anodyne, cholagogue, bitter tonic.
Indications	White poplar is an excellent remedy to use in the treatment of arthritis and rheumatism where there is much pain and swelling. In this area, its use is quite similar to willow. It is most effective when used as part of a broad therapeutic approach and not by itself. It is very helpful during a flare-up of rheumatoid arthritis. As a cholagogue, it can be used to stimulate digestion, especially stomach and liver function where there is loss of appetite. In feverish colds and in infections such as cystitis it may be considered. As an astringent, it can be used in the treatment of diarrhea.
Preparation & dosage	DECOCTION: Put 1 to 2 teaspoons of the dried bark in a cup of water, bring to a boil and simmer for 10 to 15 minutes. Strain and drink 3 times a day. To stimulate appetite, drink 30 minutes before meals. TINCTURE: Take ½ teaspoon 3 times a day.

WILD CHERRY BARK   *Prunus serotina*

Part used	Dried bark.
Actions	Antitussive, expectorant, astringent, nervine, antispasmodic.
Indications	While this herb is not a direct relaxing remedy, it may be used for easing stress or tension induced by coughing or asthma. Due to its powerful sedative action on the cough reflex, wild cherry bark finds its main use in the treatment of irritating coughs and thus has a role in the treatment of bronchitis and whooping cough. It can be used with other herbs in the control of asthma. It must be remembered, however, that the inhibition of a cough does not equate with the healing of a chest infection, which will still need to be treated. It may also be used as a bitter where digestion is sluggish. The cold infusion of the bark may be helpful as a wash in cases of inflammation of the eyes.
Preparation & dosage	INFUSION: Pour 1 cup of boiling water onto 1 to 2 teaspoons of the dried bark and leave to infuse for 10 to 15 minutes. Drink 3 times a day. TINCTURE: Take 1 to 2 ml of the tincture 3 times a day.

WILD LETTUCE   *Lactuca virosa*

Part used	Dried leaves.
Actions	Nervine, anodyne, hypnotic, antispasmodic.

Indications   The latex of the wild lettuce was at one time
sold as "lettuce opium," naming the use of
this herb quite well! It is a valuable remedy
for use in insomnia, restlessness, and excitabil-
ity (especially in children) and other manifes-
tations of an overactive nervous system. As an
antispasmodic it can be used as part of a holistic treatment of whooping cough and dry irritated coughs in general. It will relieve colic
pains in the intestines and uterus and so may
be used in dysmenorrhea. It will ease muscular pains related to rheumatism.

Preparation   INFUSION: Pour 1 cup of boiling water onto
& dosage   1 to 2 teaspoons of the leaves and let
infuse for 10 to 15 minutes. Drink 3 times
a day. TINCTURE: Take 1 to 2 ml of the tincture 3 times a day.

WILLOW   *Salix* spp.

Part used   Bark.

Actions   Analgesic, anti-inflammatory, antipyretic,
astringent, tonic.

Indications   Willow is an ancient remedy that has been
used in various forms for rheumatism, gout,
fevers, and aches and pains of all kinds. It is
often considered to be the natural form of
aspirin. However, as described elsewhere, this
is not strictly true. It can be taken internally
for arthritic complaints and gout, headaches,
fever due to common colds or influenza, and
as an aid in treating mild diarrhea, general

neuralgia, and hay fever. Applied externally, a poultice or fomentation can be used to ease the pain of arthritic joints and as a wash for sores and burns.

Preparation INFUSION: Pour 1 cup of boiling water onto 1
& dosage to 2 teaspoons of the dried herb and leave to infuse for 10 to 15 minutes. Strain and drink 3 times a day. TINCTURE: Take ½ teaspoon 3 times a day.

WOOD BETONY   *Betonica officinalis*

Names Bishopswort, betony, Stachys betonica.

Part used Dried aerial parts.

Actions Nervine, bitter.

Indications Betony gently tones and strengthens the nervous system while it also has a relaxing action. It is used in the treatment of nervous debility associated with anxiety and tension. It will ease headaches and neuralgia when they are of nervous origin, but especially those caused by hypertension.

Combinations For the treatment of nervous headache it combines well with skullcap. In hypertensive headaches, use in combination with appropriate hypotensives.

Preparation INFUSION: Pour 1 cup of boiling water onto 1
& dosage to 2 teaspoons of the dried herb and leave to infuse for 10 to 15 minutes. Drink 3 times a day. TINCTURE: Take 2 to 6 ml of the tincture 3 times a day.

From a therapeutic perspective, the basic way to use herbs is to take them internally since it is from within that healing takes place. The ways to prepare internal remedies are numerous, but with all of them it is essential to prepare carefully to ensure you end up with a medicine that works.

Teas

There are two ways to prepare teas: as infusions or decoctions. There are some basic rules of thumb for choosing which method to use with what herb, but as with all generalizations, there are many exceptions.

Infusions are usually appropriate for non-woody material such as leaves, flowers, and some stems.

Decoctions are usually required if the herb contains any hard or woody material such as roots, bark, or nuts. The denser the plant or the individual cell walls, the more energy is needed to extract cell content into the tea, thus explaining the value of decocting. An important exception would be a root rich in a volatile oil such as valerian. The woodiness of valerian root would suggest decocting, but if the roots were simmered, the therapeutically important volatile oil would boil off.

To Make an Infusion

- Take a china or glass teapot that has been warmed and put about 1 teaspoonful of the dried herb or herb mixture into it for each cup of tea.

- Pour a cup of boiling water in the pot for each teaspoonful of herb and then put the lid on. Steep for ten to fifteen minutes. Infusions may be taken hot, which is normally best for a medicinal herb tea, cold, or even iced. They may be sweetened with licorice root, honey, or brown sugar. Any aromatic herb should be infused in a pot that has a tightly fitting lid to ensure that only a minimum of volatile oil is lost through evaporation.

Herbal tea bags can be made by filling little muslin bags with herbal mixtures, taking care to remember how many teaspoonsful have been put into each bag. They can be used in the same way as ordinary tea bags.

To Make a Decoction

- Put 1 teaspoonful of dried herb or 3 teaspoons of fresh material into a pot or saucepan for each cup of water. Dried herbs should be powdered or broken into small pieces, while fresh material should be cut into small pieces. If large quantities are made, use 1 ounce of dried herb for each pint of water. The container should be glass, ceramic, or earthenware. If using metal, it should be enameled.

- Add the appropriate amount of water to the herbs.

- Bring to a boil and simmer for the time given for the mixture or specific herb, usually ten to fifteen minutes.

If the herb contains volatile oils, cover the pot with a tight-fitting lid.

- Strain the tea while still hot.

Tinctures

In general, alcohol is a better solvent than water for plant constituents. Mixtures of alcohol and water dissolve nearly all the relevant ingredients of an herb and at the same time the alcohol acts as a preservative. Alcohol preparations are called tinctures, a word that is occasionally also used for preparations with a glycerin or vinegar base, as described below. The method given below for the preparation of tinctures shows a simple and general approach; when tinctures are prepared professionally according to descriptions in a pharmacopoeia, specific water/alcohol proportions are used for each herb, but for general use, such details are unnecessary. For home use, it is best to take an alcohol of at least 30 percent (60 proof), vodka for instance, as this is about the weakest alcohol/water mixture with a long-term preservative action.

To Make an Alcohol-Based Tincture

- Put 4 ounces of finely chopped or ground dried herb into a container that can be tightly closed. If fresh herbs are used, twice the amount should be used.
- Pour 1 pint of 30 percent (60 proof) vodka on the herbs and close tightly.
- Keep the container in a warm place for two weeks and shake it well twice every day.
- After decanting the bulk of the liquid, pour the residue into a muslin cloth suspended in a bowl.

- Wring out all the liquid. The residue makes excellent compost.
- Pour the tincture into a dark bottle. It should be kept well-stoppered.

As tinctures are stronger than infusions or decoctions, the dosage to be taken is much smaller, depending on the herb. Tinctures may be used in a variety of ways. They can be taken straight, mixed with water, or they can be added to a cup of hot water. If this is done, the alcohol will largely evaporate, leaving most of the extract in the water and possibly making the water cloudy, as resins and other constituents not soluble in water will precipitate. Some drops of the tincture may be added to a bath or footbath, used in a compress, or mixed with oil and fat to make an ointment.

Another form of alcohol-based medicine is the liquid extract, also known as a fluid extract. It is much more concentrated than tinctures with one part by volume of the fluid extract being equivalent to one part by weight of the herb.

Another way of making an alcohol-based preparation is to infuse herbs in wine. Even though wine-based preparations do not have the shelf life of tinctures and are not as concentrated, they can be both pleasant to take and effective.

To Make a Glycerin-Based Tincture

Tinctures based on glycerin have the advantage of being milder on the digestive tract and do not involve the problems associated with alcohol abuse. However, they have the disadvantage of not dissolving resinous or oily materials as well. As a solvent, glycerin is generally better than water but not as good as alcohol.

To make a glycerin tincture, make up 1 pint of a mixture consisting of one part glycerin and one part water; add 4 ounces of the dried ground herb and leave it in a well-stoppered container for two weeks, shaking it daily. After two weeks, strain and press or wring the residue as with alcoholic tinctures. For fresh herbs, due to their greater water content, put 8 ounces into a mixture of 75 percent glycerin/ 25 percent water.

Dry Preparations

Sometimes it is more appropriate to take herbs in a dry form, such as in capsules or tablets. There may be an advantage to this as the taste of the herb can be avoided, and the whole herb may be taken, including the woody material. There are, however, a number of drawbacks.

Because dry herbs are unprocessed, the plant constituents might not be readily available for easy absorption. During infusion, heat and water help to break down the walls of the plant cells and dissolve the constituents, a process that is not always guaranteed during the digestion process in the stomach and small intestine. When the constituents are already dissolved in liquid form, they are available a lot faster and begin their action sooner.

Taking all this into account, there are still a number of ways to use herbs in dry form. The main thing is to ensure that the herbs are powdered as finely as possible. This guarantees that the cell walls are largely broken down and aids digestion and absorption of the herb. Techniques used to grind the herb fine enough will also cause much heat generation through friction, which may lead to a change in chemistry. This change is usually an inappropriate one.

Capsules

The easiest way to take dry powdered herbs internally is to use gelatin capsules. Capsules not made of animal products are also available. The size needed depends on the amount of herbs prescribed per dose, the density of the plant, and the volume of the material. A capsule size 00 holds about 0.5 grams (⅛ ounce) of finely powdered herb.

- Place the powdered herbs in a flat dish and take the halves of the capsule apart.
- Move the halves of the capsules through the powder, filling them in the process.
- Push the halves together.

Pills

There are a number of ways to make pills, depending on the degree of technical skill you possess. The simplest way to take an unpleasant-tasting remedy is to roll the powder into a small pill with fresh bread, which works most effectively with herbs such as goldenseal or cayenne.

- Grind herbs as fine as possible (a coffee grinder works well).
- Add a small amount of water and maple syrup to make a mud pie consistency.
- Knead slippery elm powder in a bit of bread to roll into small balls.

Baths

A pleasant way to absorb herbal compounds through the skin is to take a full body bath with 1 pint of an infusion or decoction added to the water. Any herb that can be taken internally can also be used in a bath. Herbs can, of course, also be used to give the bath an excellent fragrance.

Appendix

Actions of Herbs

ADAPTOGENS increase resistance and resilience to stress, enabling the body to avoid collapse by adapting to the problem. Adaptogens appear to work through support of the adrenal glands.

ALTERATIVES gradually restore proper functioning of the body, increasing health and vitality. Some alteratives support natural waste elimination via the kidneys, liver, lungs, or skin. Others stimulate digestive function or are antimicrobial.

ANTICATARRHALS help the body remove excess mucus, whether in the sinus area or other parts of the body. Catarrh is not of itself a problem, but when too much is produced, it is usually in response to an infection or excess carbohydrate in the body.

ANTI-INFLAMMATORIES soothe inflammations or reduce the inflammation of the tissue directly. They work in a number of different ways but rarely inhibit the natural inflammatory reaction as such; rather, they support and encourage the work the body is undertaking.

ANTIMICROBIALS help the body destroy or resist pathogenic microorganisms. They help the body strengthen its own resistance to infective organisms and throw off the illness. While some contain chemicals that are antiseptic or specific poisons to certain organisms, in general they aid the body's natural immunity.

ANTISPASMODICS ease cramps in muscles. They alleviate muscular tension and, as many are also nervines, ease psychological tension as well. There are antispasmodics that reduce muscle spasms throughout the body and also those that work on specific organs or systems.

ASTRINGENTS have a binding action on mucous membranes, skin, and other tissue, due to chemicals called *tannins*. They have the effect of precipitating protein molecules, thus reducing irritation and inflammation, creating a barrier against infection that is helpful in wounds and burns.

BITTERS are herbs with a bitter taste, with a special role in preventive medicine. The taste triggers a sensory response in the central nervous system. A message goes to the gut releasing digestive hormones leading to a range of actions including the stimulation of appetite as well as the flow of digestive juices; an aid to the liver's detoxification work; and an increased bile flow. Bitters also stimulate gut self-repair mechanisms.

CARDIAC REMEDIES have a beneficial action on the heart. Some of the remedies in this group are powerful cardioactive agents such as foxglove, whereas others are gentler, safer herbs such as hawthorn and motherwort.

CARMINATIVES are rich in aromatic volatile oils that stimulate the digestive system to work properly and with ease, soothing the gut wall, reducing any inflammation that might be present, easing gripping pains, and helping to remove gas from the digestive tract.

DEMULCENTS are rich in mucilage that soothes and protects irritated or inflamed tissue. They reduce irritation down the whole length of the bowel, reduce sensitivity to potentially corrosive gastric acids, help to prevent diarrhea, and reduce the muscle spasms that cause colic. They also ease coughing by soothing bronchial tension and relax painful spasm in the bladder.

DIAPHORETICS promote perspiration, helping the skin eliminate waste from the body, thus helping the body ensure a clean and harmonious inner environment. Some produce observable sweat, while others aid normal background perspiration. They often promote dilation of surface capillaries, thus helping to improve poor circulation. They support the work of the kidneys by increasing cleansing through the skin.

DIURETICS increase the production and elimination of urine. In herbal medicine, with its ancient traditions, the term is often applied to herbs that have a beneficial action on the urinary system. They help the body eliminate waste and support the whole process of inner cleansing.

EMMENAGOGUES stimulate menstrual flow and activity. In most herbals, however, the term is used in the wider sense of a remedy that normalizes and tones the female reproductive system.

EXPECTORANTS are herbs that stimulate removal of mucus from the lungs, and they are a tonic for the entire respiratory system. Stimulating expectorants irritate the bronchioles causing expulsion of material. Relaxing expectorants soothe bronchial spasms and loosen mucus secretions, helping in dry, irritating coughs.

HEPATICS aid the liver. They tone, strengthen, and in some cases increase the flow of bile. In a broad holistic approach to health, they are of great importance because of the fundamental role of the liver in the working of the body.

HYPOTENSIVES are remedies that lower abnormally elevated blood pressure.

LAXATIVES stimulate bowel movements. Stimulating laxatives should not be used long term. If this appears to be necessary, then diet, general health, and stress should all be closely considered.

NERVINES help relieve the nervous system and can be meaningfully subdivided into three groups: Nervine tonics strengthen and restore the nervous system. Nervine relaxants ease anxiety and tension by soothing both body and mind. Nervine stimulants directly stimulate nerve activity.

RUBEFACIENTS generate a localized increase in blood flow when applied to the skin, helping healing, cleansing, and nourishment. They are often used to ease the pain and swelling of arthritic joints.

TONICS nurture and enliven. Truly gifts of nature to a suffering humanity, tonics are whole plants that enliven whole human bodies, gifts of the Mother Earth to her children. To ask how they work is to ask how life works!

VULNERARIES are remedies that promote wound healing. Used mainly to describe herbs for skin lesions, the action is just as relevant for inner wounds such as stomach ulcers.

Headaches

Awang, D.V.C. "Feverfew." *Pharm J* 239 (1987):487.

Bohimann, F. and C. Zdero. "Sesquiterpene lactones and other constituents from *Tanacetum parthenium*." *Phytochemistry* 21 (1982): 2643.

Chung, M.K. and D.E. Kraybill. "Headache: a marker of depression." *Journal of Family Practice* 31 (1990):360–64.

Collier, H.O.J. et al. "Extract of feverfew inhibits prostagladine biosynthesis." *Lancet* 11 (1980): 922–23.

Cutler, Robert W.P. "Headache." *Scientific American* (February 1993).

Groenewegen, W.A. "Amounts of feverfew in commercial preparations of the herb." *Lancet* 1 (1986): 44–45.

Heptinstall, S. "Feverfew—an ancient remedy for modern times." *Journal of the Royal Society of Medicine* 81 (1988): 373–74.

Heptinstall, S. et al. "Extracts of feverfew inhibit granule secretion in blood platelets and polymorphonuclear leucocytes." *Lancet* 1 (1985): 1071–74.

McIntyre, Anne. *The Complete Woman's Herbal.* New York: Henry Holt, 1994.

Murphy, J.J., S. Heptinstall, and I.R.A. Mitchell. "Randomised double-blind placebo-controlled trial of feverfew in migraine prevention." *Lancet* 11 (1988): 189–92.

Pugh, W.J. and K. Sambo. "Prostaglandin synthetase inhibitors in feverfew." *Journal of Pharmacy and Pharmacology* 40 (1988): 743–45.

Rasmussen, B.K. and J. Olesen. "Symptomatic and nonsymptomatic headaches in a general population." *Neurology* 42 (1992): 1225.

Stewart et al. "Prevalence of migraine headache in the United States. Relation to age, income, race, and other sociodemographic factors." *JAMA* 267 (1992): 64–69.

Soule, Deb. *The Roots of Healing: A Woman's Book of Herbs.* New York: Citadel Press, 1995.

Waller, P.C. et al. "Efficacy of feverfew as prophylactic treatment of migraine." *British Medical Journal* 291 (1985): 1128.

Insomnia

Ancoli-Israel, Sonia. *All I Want Is a Good Night's Sleep.* St. Louis: Mosby, 1996.

Hauri, Peter and Shirley Linde. *No More Sleepless Nights.* New York: Wiley, 1996.

Keville, Kathi. *Herbs for Health and Healing.* Emmaus, Penn.: Rodale Press, 1996.

Lark, Susan. *Easing Anxiety and Stress Naturally.* Los Angeles: Keats Publishing, 1996.

Murray, Michael. *Encyclopedia of Nutritional Supplements.* Rocklin, Calif.: Prima Publishing, 1996.

Stress

Barenboim, G. M. and N.B. Kozlova. "Use of *Eleutherococcus* extract for increasing the biological resistance of man exposed to different unfavourable environmental factors" (A Review).

Bisset, Norman G., ed. *Herbal Drugs & Phytopharmaceuticals.* Boca Raton, Fla.: CRC Press, 1994.

Brekhman, II, and O. Kirillov. "Effect of eleutherococcus on alarm-phase of stress." *Life Science* 8, no.3 (Feb. 1, 1969): 113–21.

Bourne, Edmund J. *The Anxiety and Phobia Workbook.* Oakland, Calif.: New Harbinger Publications, 1990.

Davis, Martha, Elizabeth Robbins Eshelman, and Matthew McKay. *The Relaxation and Stress Reduction Workbook.* Oakland, Calif.: New Harbinger Publications, 1988.

Grieve, Maude. *A Modern Herbal.* Volumes I and II. New York: Dover Publications, 1971.

Harrer, G. and H. Sommer. "Treatment of mild/moderate depression with hypericum," *Phytomedicine* no. 1 (1994): 3–8.

Hoffmann, David. *The Complete Illustrated Holistic Herbal.* Shaftesbury, England: Element Books, 1996.

———. *An Elder's Herbal.* Rochester: Inner Traditions, 1992.

———. *The Herbal Handbook.* Rochester: Inner Traditions, 1988.

Jacobson, Edmund. *Progressive Relaxation.* University of Chicago Press: Midway Reprint, 1974.

Keville, Kathi and Mindy Green. *Aromatherapy: A Complete Guide to the Healing Art.* Crossing Press, 1995.

Leaman, Thomas L. *Healing the Anxiety Diseases.* New York: Plenum Press, 1992.

Mason, John. *Guide to Stress Reduction.* Berkeley, Calif.: Celestial Arts, 1985.

Mills, Simon. *Dictionary of Modern Herbalism.* Rochester: Inner Traditions, 1985.

Molodozhnikova, L.M. and Feldsher Akush. *Medicinal Valerian* 53, no.1 (1988): 44–46 (Published in Russian).

Murray, Michael. *Stress, Anxiety and Insomnia.* Rocklin, Calif.: Prima Publishing, 1995.

Murray, Michael and Joseph Pizzorno. *Encyclopedia of Natural Medicine.* Rocklin, Calif.: Prima Publishing, 1990.

Riggs, Maribeth. *Natural Child Care.* New York: Harmony Books, 1989.

Ulrich, R. S. "View through a window may influence recovery from surgery." *Science* 224 (1984): 420–21.

Ulrich, R. S. and R. F. Simons. "Recovery from stress during exposure to everyday outdoor environments." *In* J. Wineman, R. Barnes, and C. Zimring, eds. The Costs of Not Knowing: Proceedings of the Seventeenth Annual Conference of the Environmental Design Research Association, Washington, D.C., 1986.

Weiss, Rudolf. *Herbal Medicine.* Portland: Medicina Biologica, 1988.

Whitemore, Bob. *Living with Stress and Anxiety: A Self-Help Guide.* Manchester University Press, 1987.

Wolman, Benjamin and George Striker, eds. *Anxiety and Related Disorders: A Handbook.* New York: Wiley, 1994.

Seeds

Abundant Life Seed
Association
P.O. Box 772
1029 Lawrence St.
Port Townsend, WA 98368

Seeds of Change
P.O. Box 15700
Santa Fe, NM 87506-5700

Herbal Products

Eclectic Institute
11231 SE Market St.
Portland, OR 97216

Gaia Herbs
62 Old Littleton Road
Harvard, MA 01451

Herbalist & Alchemist Inc.
P.O. Box 553
Broadway, NJ 08808
1-800-851-5444

HerbPharm
347 East Fork Road
Williams, OR 97544

Herbs Etc.
1340 Ribina Circle
Santa Fe, NM 87501

Nature's Way Products
10 Mountain Springs
Parkway
P.O. Box 2233
Springville, UT 84663

Rainbow Light
Nutritional Systems
207 McPherson St.
Santa Cruz, CA 95060

Simpler's Botanical
P.O. Box 39
Forestville, CA 95436

Traditional Medicinal Herb
Tea Company
Sebastopol, CA 95472

Wind River
P.O. Box 3876
Jackson, WY 83001

Bulk Herbs

Blessed Herbs
109 Barre Plains Road
Oakham, MA 01068

Frontier Cooperative Herbs
Box 299
Norway, IA 52318

Mountain Rose
P.O. Box 2000
Redway, CA 95560

Trinity Herbs
P.O. Box 199
Bodega, CA 94992

Pacific Botanicals
4350 Fish Hatchery Road
Grants Pass, OR 97527

INDEX